Recalled To Life

Christopher's story

MYRTLE YEOMAN

First published in Great Britain 1995
by Alderney Books, London SW1V 9ES

The author has asserted her moral rights
ISBN 1 900253 00 3

Typeset and designed by Tangent Graphics, London N16 0DP
Printed and bound by Biddles Limited
Guildford, Surrey GU1 1DA

Profits from this book will be donated to: HEADWAY
7, King Edward Court, King Edward St, Nottingham NG1 1EW

'It's not long you see . . . say that my answer was, recalled to life.'

A Tale of Two Cities
Charles Dickens

To Guy, Patrick and Hilary, with love and thankfulness.

Contents

Introduction

My first impression of *Recalled to Life* was that it was the remarkable story of the determination of one woman and her family to do everything possible to care for and promote the recovery of her brain injured son. There is, however, another dimension to this book. It is also a significant scientific document, a record which I think is probably unique of the processes by which a person can emerge from what is called the 'persistent vegetative state' to return after a long absence to the human world of emotional relationships and intellectual life.

To permit readers to get some sense of this I propose in this introduction to discuss Christopher's story in the context of current understanding of the causes and prognosis of severe brain injury. My starting point is an article in the Lancet published in 1972, almost three years after Chris' accident — the timing we will see is important — by Bryan Jennet of the Institute of Neurological Sciences in Glasgow and Fred Plum of the Cornel Medical Centre in New York City. It is called 'Persistent Vegetative State after Brain Damage — a syndrome in search of a name'.

The authors pointed out that over the previous twenty years two events had come together to produce what was in effect a new medical problem. The first was the rising number of road traffic injuries consequent on the increase in vehicle traffic resulting in severe brain injuries to adults and children. The second was the increasing sophistication of life prolonging techniques concentrated in Intensive Care Units.

These brain injured patients thus survived when previously

they would have died. Some regained consciousness and made a good recovery, others were left with degrees of disability ranging from moderate to severe. But one group — which was their particular concern — emerged from a coma to a state of wakefulness, but without detectable awareness. There were periods during the day when their eyes were open, while at other times they might appear to be asleep. With the eyes open, they might blink but were not attentive and did not follow the movements of people or objects. They could not move their limbs voluntarily though they could make reflex movements to a painful stimulus. They were silent and neither spoke nor made any meaningful response to the spoken word. These patients were thus 'awake' without being 'aware' and could persist in this state for months or even years.

They did not require the use of a life support machine as the parts of the brain that controlled the functioning of the heart and lungs continued to function. There could be no doubt however that the higher brain functions no longer worked. This might have been due to extensive damage to the part of the brain involved in consciousness or to damage to the brain stem, through which messages pass down from the brain to the rest of the body and sensory information is co-ordinated and transmitted back upward.

Bryan Jennet and Fred Plum pointed out that this syndrome of damage had many different names — brain death, persistent, irreversible or prolonged coma, stupor or dementia, or decorticate state, all of which were unsatisfactory for one reason or another.

They proposed instead that it should be called the 'Persistent Vegetative State' because the distinguishing feature of patients with this syndrome was not the type of brain injury which they had sustained but rather their behaviour which fulfilled the Oxford English Dictionaries definition of 'vegetate' — 'to live a merely physical life, devoid of intellectual activity or social interests.'

This term has been criticized for being derogatory and dehumanising and perhaps an alternative might have been preferable but that is the one in current use and so I will continue to use it.

The importance of Jennet and Plum's article was that they gave a name to this syndrome and this was an enormous step forward. It is difficult perhaps to appreciate why, but it is necessary to imagine how prior to their article the nature and extent of this type of brain injury was not generally recognised. Thus it was difficult to investigate what form of therapies might be appropriate and to give some form of prognosis.

I emphasise this point because it both clarifies the doctor's reaction to Christopher's injuries and makes Myrtle Yeoman's determination all the more impressive. With everything we have learnt about PVS over the last twenty years, we now know that a minority of patients do indeed make some sort of recovery. But Christopher's accident occurred three years before the Lancet article appeared, so at the time the medical profession was essentially unaware of this. They believed that the prognosis of someone in Christopher's condition was hopeless and that besides providing basic nursing care until the inevitable demise there was nothing else to be done. There was certainly no inkling that the condition might be treatable, the recovery aided and accelerated by the same sort of loving care and attention that Christopher was to receive over the following years.

The key passage in this book therefore occurs at the beginning of Chapter 4. 'The doctors were kind but devastating in their frankness. They told us to have no expectations of his recovery as he had received severe injury involving the brain stem . . . My logical mind had to accept the prognosis but, curiously, as I stood by Christopher's bed, I was filled with a certainty that he would not die, and that the crucial thing was to save his mind.' In this Myrtle Yeoman's instincts were to prove more accurate than the considered judgement of the doctors with their years of experience, and this determination to trust her instincts is an essential theme of the book.

The type of brain injury Christopher sustained was almost certainly a shearing of the nerve cells and their connection to the brain stem. As I have already mentioned this is the 'highway' of the brain which messages pass up and down. The higher brain functions may be relatively intact but they are disconnected from the senses and can no longer transmit their impulses to the rest of the body.

Besides direct damage to the nerves themselves, the function of others in close proximity are impaired by swelling of the surrounding tissues which is an immediate reaction to trauma of any kind and the beginning of the attempts by the tissues to heal themselves. Over a period of several weeks this swelling subsides, leading in turn to the recovery of function of the nerves that were not directly damaged and simultaneously there comes a variable degree of recovery of physical and mental abilities. Thus it is that out of 100 patients with PVS around 46 will show some degree of improvement over a period of six months. After this time however recovery of consciousness is very rare, only ever having been recorded in a handful of patients.

The first sign of Christopher's return of consciousness — the incident of the screw top bottle — did not occur until eight and a half months after his accident. Such a recovery, as I have said is very unusual. and twenty years ago it virtually never occurred. Why did it happen? It may partly have been due to the natural repair of the nerves themselves regrowing and making new connections in the brain stem. Alternatively it is now believed that this process can be aided by a rich and stimulating environment. Without doubt a stimulating environment encourages the maturation of a child's nervous system, so why would the same not be true for someone with PVS? This possibility was first put forward in a letter to the Lancet from two doctors attached to the Institute For Human Potential in Pennsylvania in 1978 — nine years after Christopher's accident.

As is made abundantly clear Myrtle Yeoman provided just

this sort of stimulating environment for Christopher almost from the beginning and this was her second remarkable achievement. Not only did she believe he would survive when the best of medical opinion suggested otherwise but the methods she adopted to promote that recovery were a decade ahead of their time.

Myrtle Yeoman's inspiration was a Polish prisoner of war she had met while a nurse in the Second World War. Somehow he had managed to preserve his personality through the horrors of years in a concentration camp and when she asked him how he had survived, she tells us, 'He replied "I used my memories"'. Then she adds 'With these few words, the key to my approach to my son's catastrophe was put into my hands, even before he was born.'

Later on Myrtle Yeoman describes the therapeutic philosophy inspired by the Polish prisoner of war. 'I felt keenly that the key to unlock his unconscious mind might be found in our mutual love which might be able to reach depths in his subconscious mind that were unattainable by any other means. It seemed to me that some faint spark might possibly be fanned into life by the recognition of my familiar voice and presence. I believed these messages to the senses should be strong and repetitive and insistent. But because his condition was so vulnerable, their strength would have to be found in the depth of their meaning and the associations which they would have for Chris — and so I told the family stories which had meant so much to him from childhood.'

Christopher's at times dreadfully slow but steady recovery is a glorious vindication of Myrtle Yeoman's pioneering technique — the first smile, the thumb movements to indicate 'yes' or 'no', his development of mirror writing on his chest with his thumb and so on.

Controversy continues about the precise degree that stimulation aids PVS — but there can be no doubt that without it Chris would never have been able to achieve the full intellectual potential of his damaged brain.

I suggested at the beginning that *Recalled To Life* was a significant scientific document and now I return to that point. Bryan Jennet and Fred Plum made a major contribution to medical knowledge by identifying and labelling the syndrome of PVS. Similarly Myrtle Yeoman in writing this book has contributed enormously to our knowledge of the sort of quality of life that can be achieved even in the most severely disabled of those who emerge from PVS. She has also taught us, by her own example, the means by which this can be achieved.

Dr James Le Fanu
London, 1995

Author's Note

There cannot be a parent in the land who has not entertained the awful thought that one evening their child might not come home, that one day the police would knock at their door. There is scarcely an edition of a newspaper or a television news programme which does not contain some dark shadow of this sort, often mentioned once and never referred to again.

Of all such personal tragedies, one of the hardest to bear is the sudden, long-term unconsciousness of a loved one — whether from a stroke, or perhaps an anaesthetic accident or some sudden trauma, such as a swimming or horse-riding accident. But surely the most common of all, especially amongst the young and strong, must be the never-ending carnage on our roads. No section of the population is so exposed to this as young men on motorcycles.

Where there is terrible bodily damage the surgeon, with all the resources of a modern hospital at his command, will set to work and the consequences will polarise, either as recovery or death. But with the long-term unconscious there is neither life nor death. Where the damage is to the brain, loved ones are denied on the one hand thanksgiving, and on the other, the formal rites of death. But I believe there is a role that only they can play.

For some years it has been recognised as helpful to the recovery of a child if the mother is involved in his care in hospital. In my opinion this is true with a brain-injured child or adult. The unique bond of love between the unconscious patient and the ones most dear can, I believe, reach into the depths of the unconscious mind in a way that is not accessible by any other means. A familiar reassurance is communicated, so that when the first flickering awareness returns it can be fanned and encouraged into life.

My family and I were destined to make this dreadful journey, chosen by fate to endure the unendurable. We had to do this, as it were, *in vacuo* — there was no person, no authority, no recorded wisdom to offer us help or hope. The 'valley of the shadow' through which we passed was unique, and surely worthy of record.

This book *is* that record, and it is written in the belief and earnest hope that it may offer some kind of succour to those who have to follow us, and some insights to those who are so blessed as to avoid this searing test.

Chapter One

Tragedy Strikes

It was about half-past eight on a summer's evening that tragedy changed our lives. On Thursday, 14th August, 1969, my husband and I were in the garden of our Hertfordshire home, collecting washing from the line. To this day, as I gather in sweet smelling clothes, I am transported back to the moment when I heard my daughter Hilary's frightened call that two policemen were at the door.

With a fearful premonition I knew that it was to tell of an accident to our nineteen year old son, Christopher, coming home from work on his motor bike. Such fell blows can come out of a clear sky shattering the seemingly secure foundations of anyone's life, sweeping away all one's sense of order and control. You are left stunned, emotionally helpless and floundering, engulfed by the condition described so poignantly by Francis Thompson: "when so sad, thou canst not sadder".

Yet in retrospect I can remember being so practical, as though my mind was split on two levels. Almost without thinking we gathered our night things together and, with two close friends who came as companions to support our other son Patrick and our daughter Hilary, we left for the hospital. We had been told that he had been too seriously injured to be admitted to our local hospital, and so had been taken to the Whittington Hospital at Highgate, in north London, about twelve miles away, where there was a neurosurgical unit of international renown.

When we arrived at the hospital, a large Victorian building with which we were to become so familiar over the next nine months, we were asked to wait for Christopher to be brought to the intensive care ward from the operating theatre, where an emergency operation was being performed to relieve pressure from a blood clot on his brain. Hospital waiting rooms and the long echoing corridors leading to pristine wards seem soulless and strike a chill in already fearful minds. We found that the atmosphere enhanced our apprehensive state, making us worry that any noise, even a whisper, might cause offence.

As we stood around the bed to which we had been led, I simply could not believe that the near-death prone figure, surrounded by the medical paraphernalia of drips, oxygen cylinders, monitoring screen and urine-collecting bag could possibly be our son. He was scarcely recognisable: his face was white, swollen and mask-like, his head swathed in bandages. How could it be the same vibrant boy we had seen that morning, leaving the house with his cheery, 'Bye, see you tonight,'?

I dared not touch him, he was so perilously close to death. The part of him I could best recognise was his feet, and these I felt a compulsion to stroke. My mind and body were numb and I could not look at or speak to the others. We all stood frozen by his bed, shocked beyond measure.

And what had we to say to each other? Nothing that all of us had not already agonised on in our thoughts. In times of great danger or anxiety each has to fight in his own way the battle to control and overcome his fears; no one can help, however close and however loving; it is a lonely struggle. Tears are of no use. None of us shed a single tear that night. It was almost three months before I first shed tears, and then they were not shed in sorrow for Chris, but because I was overcome with a dreadful sense of disappointment in my plans for handling his nursing.

Anxiously we made our way to the doctor's room. Kindly but gravely, the surgeon assured us that everything possible had been done and that only time would reveal the extent of the brain damage. Christopher was critically ill: we would have to wait for him to recover consciousness, and we should stay near the hospital in case we were needed during the night.

At last I realised that this was no dream, but a waking nightmare. As we stood by Christopher's bed I had an utter conviction that he would live, but from that moment I also knew that our lives would be completely altered and that I would need all my strength for the fight to save his mind. As a family we had reached a watershed. My husband Guy and I were united in a determination that this terrible event should not destroy the lives of our other children too. Our essential and immediate task was to tackle the agony and the grinding day-to-day toil of restoring to Patrick and Hilary a confident and secure base on which they could found their futures. But we knew that only if they were totally confident that we would give unstintingly to Chris all the love and caring of which we were capable could that sure foundation be laid.

Chapter Two

Catching Up With The Past

It is often said that the most formative years of our lives are those of early childhood. Because I believe this to be a fundamental truth, I will spend a little time describing Christopher's early years.

Our children had the great blessing of being brought up in Tanganyika, now Tanzania. The primaeval majesty of east Africa, the beauty of its landscape and the cheerful and resourceful dignity of its people taught us all deep and lasting values, and a special measure of self-reliance. After Chris' accident, the treasures of those early experiences were used by me in the vivid word-pictures that I was able to recall for him. By the gentle reiteration of those childhood memories — the events, influences and loving family support that helped shape his personality — I believe I was able to massage his poor numbed brain back to life. There was a wealth of material for me to draw on: so much adventure was crammed into his first twelve years.

Some years before Christopher was born, when Guy and I started our married life in Egypt, we were told that if a traveller drank of the waters of the Nile, an irresistible spell would be cast, compelling him to return. A similar charm must induce the poignant longing for Africa that afflicts anyone who has lived in that capricious continent. Our family was deeply affected; it only takes a moment for each of us to be returned in imagination to that most evocative of lands.

The influences which brought us there were sown in the early years of the Second World War. Guy was a student at the Royal

Veterinary College in London when the war broke out. He joined the army, gained a commission, and in 1942 was offered the chance of secondment to the King's African Rifles in Kenya, to take part in raising a native division for the war against Japan in Burma. Africa won his heart, and he determined that when he had completed his veterinary studies after the war, he would return.

I had spent the war years nursing, the first four years at University College Hospital in London, where I did my training to become a State Registered Nurse. The close friendships that were forged there were, thirty years later, to prove vital in my fight to save Chris. When I had qualified I went to France as a nursing sister with the Queen Alexandra's Imperial Nursing Service. All the tented hospitals were set up near Bayeux, on the Normandy bridgehead, after the D-Day landings. Later, I was given the opportunity of joining a small 100-bed detachment which could be temporarily attached to forward hospitals as the need arose. In this way we travelled through France, Belgium and Holland with General Montgomery's 21st Army Group, and just before the end of the European conflict, crossed into Germany.

This was the first time that I had ever travelled abroad: there was so much that was interesting and exciting and we were deeply conscious of being involved in living history. As nurses we were made much of, flattered and thoroughly enjoyed ourselves, but there was a deeply serious side to our lives: we would have been poor things indeed if we had not responded to the agony and tragedy of war. Some of those experiences were so deeply etched into my heart that they cannot be forgotten, and yet now I can say that I am thankful for them. The inspiration which I gained in witnessing how the most desperate conditions could be transformed, if they were faced with courage and dignity, influenced the way in which I handled Christopher's nursing care.

It was during the war, too, that I began to understand how

vital it was to keep the intellect alive, how a mind without intelligence created only a living death. That lesson was learned from nursing victims from one of Hitler's most notorious concentration camps, Belsen, and most especially from one outstanding survivor, who was a shining proof of that truth.

Just before the end of the war in Europe in 1945, the army hospital in which I was serving moved into Germany, to the town of Cleves. As the concentration camps began to be overrun, some of the victims, on the point of death, too starved and ill to be moved any distance, were admitted to my ward. By dint of careful nursing some of them were helped towards both physical and mental recovery, but many of them had had their minds so affected by starvation and their terrible experiences that they were totally withdrawn, confused and uncommunicative. The patients whom I nursed were from Poland and Yugoslavia. This created an additional problem, because none of us could speak their language.

There was one survivor, a Pole, whom I shall always particularly remember. Although he was just a living skeleton, it was the intelligence in his eyes which set him apart, and he had too, a dignity and pride that so many of his companions had lost. He knew a little English and with some difficulty taught me a few simple phrases of Polish, so that I was at least able to greet my patients in their own tongue. His gentle good manners and stoicism struck such a contrast with the other wretched souls, that I eventually asked him how it was that he had been able to preserve his personality through times of such trauma and anguish. He replied, quite simply, 'I used my memories'. With these few words, the key to my approach to my son's catastrophe was put into my hands, even before he was born.

Late in 1945 I was transferred from Germany to Egypt, to a hospital just outside Alexandria. Meanwhile Guy had returned to England from Burma, where his East African Division had been involved in the campaign against the Japanese. With ingenuity he managed to arrange a posting to Egypt, where he and

I were united after a separation of four years. Six weeks later we were married at the little English church at Abassieh, and we set up our first home in Heliopolis, the desert suburb of Cairo. In July of that year we finally came back together to Britain by troopship for demobilisation. Spirits were high at the thought of getting back to civilian life, albeit tempered with some anxiety about the uncertainties to be faced over jobs and housing.

Guy went back to the Royal Veterinary College, spending the last two years of his course at the college field station at Streatley in Berkshire. This village is on one of the most lovely stretches of the River Thames: we were young and in love and it entirely suited our mood. Because of the housing shortage in those early post-war years, we decided to investigate the possibility of buying some kind of boat and living on the river. The winter of 1946-47 was one of the most severe for centuries, and it was really no time to hunt for boats. But we were filled with a longing that was only satisfied when we discovered the Thames Sailing Barge *Murston*, a lovely old trading vessel, which was destined to be our home for the next two years. We brought her upstream from Caversham, where she was lying, and moored her alongside a little island belonging to Moulsford Manor, two miles above Streatley. And so it was that our Christopher was conceived aboard this lovely boat, a fitting ending to our idyll on the river.

On 10th September 1949 Christopher Guy was born at University College Hospital my old hospital in London. By this time my husband had qualified as a veterinary surgeon and his long held plans to return to work in Africa began to bear fruit with his appointment by the Colonial Office to the Veterinary Department in Tanganyika. It was obvious to both of us that it would be wise for him to go ahead, so that he could deal with the problems of a new job and setting up our new home. At the end of 1949 he travelled out up the Nile route by flying boat.

When Christopher was three months old, we travelled by sea to join Guy. The steamship passage to Mombasa in Kenya took a leisurely and pleasant three weeks. From my experienced fellow travellers I picked up a good deal of advice about living in the tropics — a useful initiation into our new life, and reassuring to those of us who knew we were going to remote stations, where we should be thrown upon our own resources.

Guy's first posting in Tanganyika was to the tiny outpost of Korogwe in the north-east of the country, and it was there that he had made our new home ready for us. My first sight of Tanganyika was on the journey south from Mombasa as we travelled by Land Rover over the red dust bush track to the little port of Tanga. At the time this was an unusual route — most people would have continued to Tanga by sea — but my husband was impatient to show me our adopted country, and the journey by this wild bush track, red as terracotta, with arbours of huge blue convolvulus, was a starkly beautiful introduction.

We quickly adapted to the strange conditions, revelling in the new experiences and adventures, but after only a few months we were transferred to the opposite quarter of the territory, to the Southern Highlands Province. Frequent changes of station were the lot of the vets in those days — a reflection of the continuing battle against rinderpest, a virulent and internationally known cattle disease. However, against the trend, we were destined to spend nearly seven years in this home, 6000 feet up in the south-western quarter of the territory. This was a true *home,* not just a house to live in (as so many government quarters were) and the earliest memories imprinted on our children's minds must relate to this magical place. I am sure that it was our life here that had the greatest influence on their personalities.

The house was part of a totally isolated government stock farm set deep in a characteristic type of east African open woodland called *miombo,* about a mile from the earth road that was said to run from the Cape to Cairo. The nearest township to the north was Iringa, about twenty-five miles away, and 200 miles to the south, Mbeya, near the northern Rhodesian (now Zambian) border. Our immediate neighbours were almost entirely natives of the splendid Wahehe tribe; our nearest European neighbours lived six miles away by bush track.

Our farm was called 'Iheme'; the name rhymes with 'pay me', and it is the local Kihehe name for the corky bark tree *Erythrina tomentosa* that, with its brilliant dry-season display of flame-coloured flowers, is a striking feature of those parts. Our rambling whitewashed mud-brick bungalow, which had grown through the years with sundry additions, like Topsy, was set amongst the gnarled and twisted woodland miombo trees. An avenue of jacaranda trees led up to our door, and high smokey blue eucalyptus trees — 'blue gum trees' — towered above it, swaying in the wind against the heavenly blue sky and massive silver cumulus that are such a feature of high-altitude Africa. A lovely garden fell away in terraces from the spacious verandah, which itself was shaded by an opulent canopy of creepers: passion fruit, the golden shower of Cape honeysuckle and the grape like clusters of the mauve potato creeper.

After we had been living at Iheme for a year, Patrick, our second son, was born, my husband driving me the bone-shaking twenty-five miles to Iringa Hospital in our Land Rover in the small hours of a brilliant moonlit night. He then drove back to the farm and next day told Chris that he was going to be taken to Iringa to meet his new brother. Chris, a little over two years old, disappeared completely and only after an anxious search did Guy find him trudging back along the footpath from the dam that held the headwaters of our irrigation system. This was a fascinating place where Chris delighted in watching the water-borne wildlife, and now he was struggling to carry a rather soggy cardboard box containing a water tortoise from which he refused to be parted. These amphibious tortoises are endearing creatures, equipped with a draw-bridge type of front door with which they can close themselves off from the outside world. Imagine my consternation when Chris' four-square little figure, after staggering up the verandah steps of my hospital room, tipped the contents of the box, duck-weed and all, into the new baby's cot!

After three years we took our first leave of six months in England, and at the end of this time I stayed behind with the two boys because I was expecting our third child and had been advised by my doctor to have the delivery in London. So it was that in due course we became the parents of our daughter Hilary Jane, and when she was six weeks old we set out to rejoin Guy at Iheme, where we lived for another three years. We were spared the upheaval of a new posting because Guy was assigned to special investigatory work on East Coast Fever, a disease carried by ticks, which has a major economic effect on the east African cattle industry. This unusually long posting enabled us to provide a much more stable background for the children's early years, while at the same time giving us the opportunity of travelling widely with Guy whenever it was possible.

Chapter Three

Out Of Africa

There being no school at Iheme, I undertook the education of our children myself. It was not unusual in Tanganyika for parents to do this up to the age of seven or eight, because infant schools were only available to those living in the large population centres; but in our case, a somewhat ill-starred effort to settle Chris at the age of eight into a distant preparatory boarding school came to an end when he was taken quite seriously ill. After that I determined to undertake the education of all three of our children at our home, wherever that might be.

We were introduced to an organisation called the Parents' National Education Union, whose prime task is to help families with the schooling of their children anywhere in the world. This marvellous institution is still going strong, based in England at Ambleside in the Lake District, where postal courses are prepared and despatched each term, and from where books can be borrowed from a comprehensive library list. A detailed curriculum and daily timetable is laid down; completed written and artwork has to be posted regularly to Ambleside, whence it is as regularly returned, meticulously corrected. There is nothing sloppy or easy-going about it, and for those with determination it offers for their children a uniquely high quality primary education. In this way I was able to educate our children until we eventually had to return to England.

P.N.E.U. was founded by a remarkable Victorian woman, Charlotte Mason, who set up her own college to train teachers in her self-developed educational philosophy. This was far in advance of her time and was based on the recognition that every child has a unique personality. Pupils were to be encouraged to seek knowledge by keen observation, stimulating a lively questioning attitude. Whatever work the child produced he was to be commended, never chided or made to feel inadequate; this was always my aim, although I know I fell short of the ideal many times.

When we were at our home we used a large garage beside the house as a schoolroom, but if we were on safari, a tent or rest house was all we needed. Like a snail, I took the schoolroom on my back. I used to say to the children, 'You must realise that *I* am learning too!' And so together, we tackled this fascinating quest for knowledge. I felt that the intimate insight this gave me into the way our children's minds worked was a great privilege; it was also a tremendous help when I began to try to stimulate Chris' mind on its slow road back to awareness. Neither I nor the children have ever regretted their early home-school days: indeed, I know they consider them to have been a real advantage in their later years, and I believe it forged another important link between us.

However, there were some limitations to this do-it-yourself education. It was sometimes difficult not to get over-anxious or irritable — sometimes because you knew they were not doing as well as you felt they were capable of, sometimes because we were tired or hot. In order to break this possible build up of tension, I made it a rule that we would all be free to do whatever we wanted between midday and four in the afternoon. This was always the hottest part of the day and it seemed only sensible to adopt the Spanish custom of siesta.

Although we tackled all the subjects on the curriculum, the usual type of games played in English schools were beyond me. When we returned to Britain and Chris went to Highgate School, he brought home an impressive silver cup at the end of his first term. I was delighted, interpreting this as a tribute to my early teaching. Alas, no! It had been awarded to him as 'the most improved footballer of the year'. Small wonder — he could scarcely have known one end of a football pitch from the other when he started!

In the southern highlands region where we lived for so long, most of our European friends came from the sparsely scattered settler population, who were more noteworthy for their engaging eccentricity than for their grasp of tropical agri-business! Living in such circumstances, we naturally became very dependent upon our African staff who worked in our home and garden and on the Veterinary Department farm. They were loyal and long serving, and took their attachment to our family seriously. They were all marvellous with the children, infinitely patient and kind, with a most endearing sense of humour. This was completely disarming and had power to turn away wrath more quickly than any carefully-phrased apology.

One of our African staff was especially loved. His name was Samweli, and he came from the neighbouring Bena tribe, who inhabit the Njombe district, to the south of the Hehe country. He came to us as a garden boy when he was about fourteen years old. Through the years he advanced in our household hierarchy until he became 'major domo', which, in our little world, meant head house-boy. He married from our house and brought his bride to live in their homestead on the edge of our farm. There his children were born and brought up. When we had finished with our school books, I used to give them to Samweli so that he could educate his own family. The earliest primers I bought, before the P.N.E.U. days, were in the Kiswahili language and full of African daily situations such as 'If your mother put out three shirts on the ground to dry and a goat ate one, how many would be left?'

Samweli gave us nearly twelve years of devoted service and his exceptional personality has provided our family with a pivot upon which we can hang many of our 'Do you remember . . . ?' stories. Saying goodbye to him when we eventually left for England was the first experience our children suffered of bereavement; their homesickness as we tried to adjust to life in

Britain often related to some incident of our African life in which Samweli was involved.

Iheme was a beautiful place in which to bring up our children; there were almost no restrictions on their freedom and enjoyment of the countryside. East Africa was then a place of absolute peace and security. It was my husband's boast at Iheme that he never had a gun or even a key to the house, and never bolted a door or window at night. I believe this lifestyle bound us closely as a family, not in any suffocating sense, but by the mutual recognition of the unique qualities each could contribute in a situation where little outside help was available. I think it was this isolation that made us respect each other's individual attributes. I know that, years later, I was to be thankful for that intimate understanding between us, which proved so fundamental in helping Chris towards recovery.

We lived in harmony with our African neighbours, admiring their stoicism and adaptability. They in turn would come to me for medical help. Each day, when I was at home, I would hold an unofficial clinic, and in return, they would bring little gifts of vegetables, eggs or chickens. There was a mutual respect which was heart-warming.

This way of life made us independent and inventive. We lived entirely without the constant brain-numbing effect of newspapers, radio and television, and this led to it becoming instinctive for me to act on my own initiative, using whatever resources happened to be available. Without a telephone, and being miles from any sort of qualified help, I was thrown on my own resources. I just had to do what I thought best in the circumstances; I could not let the destructive forces of anxiety or fear dissipate my resolve or weaken my judgement. If things went wrong I had to face the consequences and argue my case. This background proved a strict but needful training-ground for the lonely decisions I had to take later in order to bring Chris through his terrible ordeal. I thank God that I had those experiences. They were the rich, vividly coloured threads that I used as the warp for Christopher's personal tapestry — the constant threads through which the others were woven.

For twelve years we lived in and travelled throughout British East Africa, which was the umbrella title for Tanganyika, Kenya and Uganda. The wind of change brought independence first to Tanganyika, under the presidency of Julius Nyerere, and in due course under the name Tanzania in 1961, and we returned to England to find a new home and start a fresh life. We all felt a deep homesickness for Africa, but eventually settled down in a lovely house backing on to the Great Wood of Northaw in southern Hertfordshire. From here the children were able to travel daily to their schools on the northern fringe of London. There were good and bad years, years of achievement, sadness, struggle and loss, but our family life proved a sure foundation for the trials we were destined to face and overcome.

During this time two or three of Christopher's attainments gave us special satisfaction. After successfully completing the Bronze and Silver Awards of the Duke of Edinburgh's Scheme, he finally achieved the Gold in 1967, and I had the great happiness of accompanying him to Buckingham Palace for his presentation from Prince Philip. The following year, he was one of seventeen boys selected for the British Schools' expedition to Spitzbergen in the Arctic, and in 1969 he was accepted by Hatfield Polytechnic (now a university) for their biology course. It was while he was doing a vacation job prior to the start of that autumn term that the dreadful accident happened, and all his and our hopes were swept away.

For months after his accident I used the fine web woven from these stories of travel and adventure to trawl the dark waters of Christopher's unconsciousness. Gradually fragments of his shattered mind were gathered, retrieved and brought to the surface. His mind was saved; my erstwhile patient from the Nazi holocaust had shown me the tool to use: Christopher's memories.

Chapter Four

Battle For The Mind

In the beginning it was thought that Christopher might recover consciousness in perhaps eight to twelve hours. He had been wearing the best crash helmet available and there was so little obvious damage, it seemed impossible to believe that he had sustained any serious injury. He had a few grazes, a cut on the chin and he had lost two of his front teeth, but no bones had been broken. I have already described our shocked reaction when we first saw him in the Intensive Care ward. His head had been shaved, his face was swollen and white like a mask; he was totally immobile and there was an airway in his mouth. A blood transfusion was already in progress. I felt frozen but a strong impulse made me place both my hands on his feet. I was afraid to touch him anywhere else in case I should hurt him further. He was obviously so delicately poised between life and death. All I could do was pray that God would fill my mind with the knowledge of what I had to do.

Although Chris was deeply unconscious there was no question of our being asked to agree to the switching-off of a respirator, as he was breathing unaided. The intravenous drips and catheters with urine-collecting bags were hanging about his bed, and his lungs were aspirated regularly by a suction machine. Apart from his breathing, his life was totally dependent on medical aids, which themselves inevitably put a physical barrier between the injured and their loved ones, enhancing feelings of anxiety and inadequacy.

As the hours of his unconsciousness extended into days, we realised that we would have to prepare for a long term upheaval in our family life. The doctors were kind but devastating in their frankness. They told us to have no expectations of his recovery as he had received severe injury involving the brain stem which is the seat of life, and the origin of consciousness. The design of the crash helmet was altered subsequently, as it was thought to predispose to such an injury.

Their grave words were really a confirmation of what I had already suspected. I knew from my training that there was no hope for him from a purely medical point of view. But equally, I knew that it was impossible for me to accept that nothing could be done, for it is not my nature to despair. If no one could advise me, then I had to follow my instincts and find a way myself. I believe that one's instincts are the inherited wisdom of the ages which can be released in moments of dire need. My logical mind had to accept the prognosis but, curiously, as I stood by Christopher's bed, I was filled with a certainty that he would not die, and that the crucial thing was to save his mind.

Much later, when I felt more confident, my instinctive reaction was to stroke him, gently reassuring him by the soft reiteration of his name that he was safe and I was Mum and would be with him always. But for now I had to allow myself to be controlled by my instincts and tap these inner resources, clearing my mind of doubts, anxieties and inhibiting pre-conceptions. In particular, I had to learn to overcome my sense of inadequacy in the face of authority and scholarship.

My attitude may have seemed misguided — even arrogant — to others. I suppose it must have been assumed that my inability to accept the bleak prognosis was due to shock. However, I could not let the opinion of others deter me. The situation was so grave that I needed all my strength — mental and physical and spiritual — to cope with it, and I could not spare any energy for regrets over what had been lost or what might have been. I knew that I would have to work with intensive effort and un-deviating concentration.

It was vitally important that I kept my mind absolutely clear and sensitively able to respond to every nuance in Chris' condition. Soon after the accident, our well-meaning family doctor sent me a supply of sleeping tablets, believing that I would need them to help me deal with the shock and despair. I flushed them safely down the lavatory.

I have never believed that tranquillisers have any place in helping people through dreadful periods of anxiety. They only fuzz the mind and, at such times, it is essential that one's judgement and imagination are kept razor-keen. Nor would I touch alcohol. The only stimulant I would take was tea — Guy must have made me gallons of that refreshing brew! At night, he would bring me a cup of warm milk and honey to help me to relax into sleep.

Day after day we would arrive at Christopher's bedside only to discover that his profoundly unconscious state was unchanged and his condition was still critical. Sheer exhaustion, desperate anxiety and the total uncertainty of the future made it almost impossible for Guy and me to sit down and think through our situation. We just didn't have the time; our minds were totally occupied with thoughts of Chris.

But all the while we knew that it was essential also to concern ourselves with the lives of our other two children, Patrick and Hilary. A cataclysmic disaster such as this affects every member of a family. Each of us had a special relationship with Chris; we had to let our children grieve in their own way but we also had to assure them that *their* lives were equally important to us. Although we had told them honestly all we knew about their brother's condition and the fears for the future, they still had their own lives to live. Our parental wish to protect them must not cause their natural need to accept life fully and adventurously to be thwarted by any sense of guilt at enjoyment or a feeling that, by accepting risk, they might be adding to our anxieties. Only if they were assured that Chris was receiving all the love and help it was possible for us to give him, would they feel free to do this. Obviously we would all be under stress, almost to breaking point.

It is difficult to describe my thoughts at this time, they were so turbulent. My emotions were so intense that I felt aware of everything with an enhanced perception. Any form of beauty filled my heart with a poignancy quite beyond words. Those memories have never left me. Anything pretentious or insincere I found abhorrent, and yet now the piercing shock has passed, I am almost shy of admitting to this self-consciousness about the depth of my emotions.

At the time of the accident Patrick was seventeen years old and Hilary fifteen. Both were studying for important examinations. How they managed to work I shall never understand, as concentration was almost impossible. They were denied the motherly attentions I longed to give them. The demands made on Guy and me were so pressing and immediate that we had little energy to discuss our problems even with each other, let alone the children. We fell naturally into a pattern whereby I would watch over Chris at the hospital and Guy would support Paddy and Hilary. Almost the only time of the day we had alone together was the brief moment or two when Guy would wake me with a cup of tea.

Although there was such relentless pressure on our every waking hour, there were certain matters which could not be overlooked. Somehow Guy had to take up his working life again. Returning from east Africa to Britain in 1961 had been a necessary sacrifice in the interests of keeping our family together while the children embarked on their secondary education. In the circumstances, my husband had thought himself lucky to obtain a post with a leading pharmaceutical research company, heading their Veterinary Clinical Research Unit in developing the recently discovered semi-synthetic penicillins for worldwide veterinary use. But this was not where his heart lay; it lay still in Africa and when, after eight years back in England, he had received an offer from the Food and Agricultural Organisation of a major assignment in his particular field of tropical cattle disease in east Africa, we had persuaded ourselves that the children were by now sufficiently settled in their education to allow this degree of separation. The attractions of the new post included annual visits by his family to Africa as well as annual leave for him in Britain. Only a few days before Christopher's accident, Guy had had his medical for the new job, and the contract awaited his signature. Most fortunately he had not anticipated this by tending his resignation to his existing employers, and after the blow fell, one of his first actions was to cancel the FAO appointment.

Now he was effectively a prisoner, for the remainder of his professional life, of work that was not his first choice — a situation, of course, in which many people find themselves. In his case it was ameliorated by the kindness of his colleagues and the helpfulness of his company, and we were truly thankful to be so fortunate as to have a sufficient and secure income over the years that followed. This enabled me, without disruption, to give the whole of my time to Chris.

For the first year Guy was able to combine being at home when Hilary and Paddy came back from school with visiting the hospital later in the evening — a complicated arrangement that required buying a second car. But unfortunately, after this first year, his work was transferred from Hertfordshire to Surrey, and this necessitated his being away for five nights a week. Kind friends who lived near her school took Hilary into their home for this period, while Paddy was taking his first independent steps as a medical student in London.

In this way we adapted as best we could to the disruption of our family life. But there was no time for listening, discussing or just being quietly together. Of all the times in life when that is of the greatest importance, I believe it to be the teenage years. All this easy companionship was denied to Patrick and Hilary. We had very good friends and cousins nearby whose help was invaluable, but this could not be the same as their own close family. I think this forced our children to develop a defensive, self-protecting skin which could have been mistaken for assured independence, but which really masked an inner loneliness and heartache. There was no way we could find the perfect solution. All we could do was to meet their needs as we became aware of them and do our best under the circumstances.

One such concern was to think of ways in which I could soften the bleakness of their return to an empty house, and make them aware of my love and concern, despite my absorption with Chris. As it was a lovely summer and the garden was ablaze with blossom, I filled the house with flowers. Later in the year, as winter approached, we bought an electric fire with simulated coals, to provide an instant glow of welcome to the dark house. Thanks to a new cooker with automatic timer the comforting smell of home cooking greeted them on their return home. All the time I felt a desperate guilt that I was neglecting them, but there seemed no other course to follow than the one we had chosen.

Every day seemed the same. There was no let-up in the incessant round of work, the endless treadmill. I felt that there was a danger that I might transmit a sense of anxiety or alarm to Chris, so I forced myself to be calm at his bedside. In an attempt to dispel this anxious state of pent up emotion, on the way to the hospital each day it became my habit to call in to rest and pray in our village church. It was marvellous to be alone in that lovely place. I was able to pour out my heart where no one could be troubled by my distress. The solace and peace that I found there soothed me. It was almost as though its ancient walls were imbued with a special quality of comfort.

But in truth the only *real* peace I knew was at the hospital with Chris. At least there I knew what was happening; away from there, I felt torn and anxious. Approaching the ward each day was an agony, as I never knew in what condition I should find him, so finely did his life hang on a thread in those early days.

To start with — for the first few weeks — Guy would telephone the hospital every morning for a report, desperately hoping that one day there might be even the slightest inflection of hope in the ward sister's voice. But never, never was this so: only the immutable 'no change . . . condition stable . . . still unconscious . . . ' Eventually, by silent tacit consent, he abandoned this practice, so from then on I faced the ward each day unarmed.

It was in the December after the accident that I felt most certain of God's help. At this time Chris was passing through a crisis of hypothermia. For ten days he suffered numerous periodic convulsions of severe rigors, accompanied by high temperatures and drenching sweats. His bed would be shaken violently as his body was engulfed by these paroxysms, and we would watch helplessly as sweat poured from his body just as though water had been thrown over him. Through all the long period of heartache we suffered, I think this caused me the greatest anguish.

One morning, towards the end of this fearful episode, I called in to our village church as I always did on the way to the hospital, but this time I broke down in passionate weeping. I felt so desolate and alone. It was the first time I had cried since the accident: I cried out in my agony to God to help me, and at once I felt my hands taken. It was as though they were gripped by a friend and I was brought up from my knees. I know that Christ was there to help and support me. From that time onwards I never doubted that God was with me. Wonderfully comforted, I left for the hospital. Even now, so many years later, the miracle of that moment remains with me.

Once I was at Christopher's bedside I thought it was important to impart reassurance to him. The clinical correctness of the neurosurgical ward struck cold fear in my heart. Logically I recognised how fortunate we were to have him there, but I was afraid that it might have the same chilling effect on any slight awareness which might be returning to Chris. I felt a compulsion to talk softly and continually to him. It was equally instinctive for me to hold his hands and stroke the most tender parts of his arms. Gradually it dawned on me that I was attempting to communicate with him by using two of our five senses, those of touch and hearing. It occurred to me that, by stimulating also the senses of sight, smell and taste, I might be able to trigger a stronger response in his mind.

I felt keenly that the key to unlock his unconscious mind might be found in our mutual love. I was certain that in a subtle way, by being with him, I helped him to relax, as though my presence comforted him. I now began to believe that my love for him might be able to reach depths in his subconscious mind that were unattainable by any other means. It seemed to me that some faint spark might possibly be fanned into life by the recognition of my familiar voice and presence. I believed these messages to the senses should be strong and repetitive and insistent. But because his condition was so vulnerable, their strength would have to be found in the depth of their meaning and the associations which they would have for Chris.

So I told the family stories which had meant so much to him from childhood. Again and again my Polish patient's words came back to me, 'I used my memories'. In order to increase the sensation of touch, I brought eau de cologne fresheners to use in my stroking and massaging; to increase their effect, I chilled them overnight in the refrigerator, bringing them to the hospital each day in a thermos flask. While I massaged the sensitive parts of his arm, and over the palms of his hands down to the tips of his fingers, I would talk softly of familiar places and friends.

With single-minded purpose I drove myself to use every means in my power to stir any emotional response in Christopher's mind. It seemed to me that if I revived memories of his early impressionable years in Africa they would have a special significance. So, with my arms cradling his head I would talk of Tanganyika and our family experiences. Sometimes, to vary the tone of the sound I would hum tunes of his childhood to him, in the way one would croon to soothe a troubled child. I always spoke gently, feeling an almost physical need to massage his poor brain with the balm of soft sound. It was only when I sensed that his brain was growing stronger that I increased the strength of my voice; at first I spoke very softly as if to a newly born child.

After three months it was necessary for Chris to be moved from the neurosurgical ward to a general ward. The consultant suggested that Chris should be put into one of the side wards to facilitate my working with him. This gave me freedom to extend my ideas. Of course, anything I did was done with the full support of the doctors and nursing staff, I could have done nothing without that. They knew how thankful we were for all the care that they gave to Chris, and they were supportive and sympathetic with my approach. They, like we, were longing for it to show results, hoping that something would break through this icy barrier of unconsciousness. Nothing I did impeded their work; rather it relieved them of the necessity of close supervision, as they knew that I would recognise and report any change in Christopher's condition, just as though I had been a member of staff.

In an effort to evoke memories for him in every possible way, I brought articles to the hospital for which I knew he had a particular fondness. One such was a much loved little African-made soap-stone elephant which he had bought with his first pocket money. It was a beautiful object, smooth and cool and small enough to fit comfortably into the palm of his hand. Later, when I thought music might be helpful, I brought our old wind-up gramophone which we had used in Africa, with a selection of his favourite records. I hoped its tinny resonance might be evocative and stir the response of nostalgia in his mind. Over and over again I played our record of *Kwa Heri,* the African farewell.

Over the weeks and months I gradually increased the time-scale of these experiences, as I felt his condition was strengthening and his mind developing. Hoping to trigger remembrance, I read much loved books of his childhood to him, such as Kenneth Grahame's *The Wind in the Willows*, the Pooh books by A.A. Milne, and the Ernest Thompson Seton wildlife stories. Being ageless in their appeal, I thought they would be of interest at whatever stage his mental recovery might have reached.

Each day I brought a fresh rose to the hospital from our garden: in our woodland situation, we had roses flowering even into December. I described to him where I had found it, hoping that its colour and sweet scent would stimulate his sight and sense of smell. Although no one believed that he could see, I thought it was important to stimulate this sense, in the same way as any of the others. My actions must have seemed ridiculous and pathetic, because all this time, several months after the accident, *he responded to nothing*, being still profoundly unconscious.

Every day when we arrived at his bedside we would glance covertly at his medical chart. The staff had a scoring system for the level of consciousness, graded from fully conscious to the deepest level of unconsciousness. Every day, as the weeks turned to months and the months drew on to make the first year, without exception we saw that he was graded at the very lowest level. But even so I was driven on by a compulsion that I simply could not deny. Perhaps it was the maternal instinct, that simply made me do everything I could to help Chris, whatever others might think. If he was going to live, I had to save his mind.

Therefore, undeterred, I brought some of Christopher's own drawings and paintings to show him. He was clever at drawing and interested in art. One drawing in particular I felt might have memories for him because he had laboured so much over it. It was of our cat, which really belonged to Chris since it was he who, on the way from school, had seen the notice in a shop window, and chosen his pick from the litter. I decided to hang it on his locker at the side of his bed. Although at this time it was thought that he could not see, and his eyes were permanently open and staring at the blank walls of the ward, I felt that, if there was any chance of returning sight, then this much-loved portrait of Puss would be comforting to him.

And so I persisted day in, day out, as interminable, meaningless time passed. The medical and nursing staff were usually kind and tolerant but always uncomprehending of my behaviour, which must have seemed completely time-wasting and misguided to them. Although numerous neurological examinations were made throughout the first three months, only the last of these was anything but hopeless. That one, an E.E.G. (electro-encephalograph) showed a pattern of brain activity which surprised his doctors by its degree of normality. Otherwise there was nothing but the grim, hopeless unresponsiveness of profound unconsciousness. I know that now many of those working with brain injured people are beginning to use various arousal techniques; but this was in 1969 and no one then could see any usefulness in my approach, believing it to be deluded effort stemming from my inability to come to terms with the hopelessness of his condition.

Chapter Five

A Glimmer Of Hope

I was able to establish a much greater closeness to Christopher than is usual in the hospital situation of visitor and patient because he was so critically ill and not expected to live. Even months after the accident his expectation of life was measured in days. Although hours of visiting were strictly limited, out of sympathy towards us the nursing and medical staff allowed me exceptional access and licence in handling Chris. They knew of course that I was a State Registered Nurse, but even so they treated me with amazing forbearance.

We had bought a second car, a Mini, and for the whole of the year I'm describing I made the double journey, ten miles each way, between our home and the hospital, every day without exception, to be joined most evenings by Guy and Patrick after school — Highgate School being only a mile up the hill from the hospital. Sadly, Hilary was not allowed into the ward because she was under sixteen. This exclusion made it more difficult for her to come to terms with what had happened and I know that it caused great unhappiness and a sense of rejection. For the first time ever she was being denied involvement in a serious family matter.

Irrespective of his unconsciousness Christopher's state of health varied considerably. I have already described the serious complications of hypothermia which he suffered about three months after the accident. This is associated with certain types of brain damage, when the temperature control mechanism goes out of control. In conjunction with these attacks, which went on over a period of ten days, he developed renal stones and bladder gravel which produced blood-stained urine. He would become flushed and then his limbs would tense as though suffering bouts of considerable pain. But he made no sound and there was no apparent change in his level of consciousness. Although it was dreadful to watch these spasms, which only ceased after he had been given Valium, it was the first sign of a reaction of any sort from him. I was told that these were complications frequently met with in long-term immobile patients who suffer a release of calcium from their bones. As no one could tell me why this occurred but only that it was always associated with total helplessness, I decided to move Chris vigorously, turning him frequently, and from that time onwards we had no recurrence of the problem.

My first inclination had been to handle Chris very delicately, disturbing him as little as possible and treating him as one would treat any seriously ill patient. But of course his problem was one of deep unconsciousness and therefore, because he was unable to move himself, I had to force activity upon him. Turning him from side to side I would massage his body to stimulate the circulation and, while holding him over the edge of the bed, carry out vigorous chest drainage to keep his lungs in as good a condition as possible. I would cup my hands so that the cushion of air trapped in their palms would spread the effect of pummelling and beating his chest, doing this rhythmically, side, back and front. He was given antibiotics continuously as a prophylactic against infection, which is an ever-present risk to anyone nursed in hospital because of the danger of cross-infection. But, after he came home, this was discontinued because I was able to keep his chest clear by this regular physiotherapy alone.

Later, when this disturbed period had passed and he had relapsed into quiescence, it occurred to me that Chris, although still unconscious, might be helped if I involved him in such simple tasks as teeth-cleaning and face-washing. I thought that these disciplines, natural between a mother and a child, might trigger a response in his subconscious mind. While holding his hand tightly round the flannel or toothbrush and making the actions slowly and deliberately, I would describe what I was doing. Because the sense of hearing is thought to be the first to return, I always felt it was very important to explain each action as it was carried out.

Gradually I increased the ways by which I could stimulate his mind and improve his exercises. Slowly I felt Chris growing stronger. About six months after his accident I noticed that the unnaturally strange and fine, almost parchment-like, quality of his skin had given way to a more normal appearance and he began to put on a little of the weight he had lost. Altogether he was looking better but still with no demonstrable change in his level of unconsciousness. For some time I had believed I could see intelligence in his eyes, and although I could detect no physical response, I sensed that he was aware of me and relaxed in my presence. Then, quite out of the blue, after eight and a half months of total unresponsiveness an incident occurred which convinced me he had the mental capacity to make an intelligent appraisal of a situation.

As I worked day after day with Chris, carrying out all the simple repetitive tasks I had devised and which by now were almost automatic, one part of my brain was keenly alert to any change I might notice in his condition. On this particular occasion, almost at the end of our usual routine, something momentous occurred. It was only a slight thing but was of such significance I could hardly bring myself to believe in it.

One of my foibles was to bring from home all the things I needed to carry out our simple routine of face-washing and mouth-cleaning. It all helped me to talk to Chris about familiar things and speak of our daily village goings-on. On this day, on my way to the hospital, I had called in to buy yet another small bottle of glycerine from our local chemist. After teeth-cleaning, one always completes the task by swabbing the lips and mouth of the long-term sick with a little glycerine. In the past weeks and months this had always come from a corked bottle. As with all these actions I tried to involve Chris by cupping his hand in mine and directing the movement to push the cork in the bottle to close it. On this day I felt a resistance and saw a slight twisting movement of his right thumb. Although this was little more than a tremor, it was the first voluntary movement he had made. Astonished I looked at our hands; our fingers held a metal cap not a cork. For the first time I had been given a *screw-capped* bottle.

Suddenly I realised that Chris had been trying to correct my thrusting movement to change it to a screwing action. This was typical of him. He had scant respect for my understanding of mechanical things. I could almost see the wry look and hear the humorous chuckle at my foolishness. It was only a tiny breach in the impassive blankness of his apparently unconscious state, but I knew that a miracle had happened; I felt quite certain that his mind had been saved. All I needed now was time, perseverance and courage. I just turned to him and threw my arms about him, hugging him while the tears ran down my cheeks.

Of course no one else had witnessed this incident. Even had they been present they would scarcely have noticed it, and since there was no question of arranging for it to be repeated, everyone else remained sceptical. But *I* knew it had happened, and felt elated.

This was a time of loneliness for us all. We had to devise our own ways of coping and coming to terms with what had happened. But of all of us I think my husband Guy found it the most difficult. He felt torn and unutterably helpless. Out of loyalty and love for me he attempted to involve himself in what I was doing at the hospital, but he was not able to believe in its real usefulness. Also he was under relentless mental pressure. Each night, after a full day's work at his research laboratory, he returned home to try to provide some kind of normality for Patrick and Hilary, and then drive up to join me at the hospital. We didn't even have each other's company for the final return journey home — usually between 10pm and 11pm — because there were two cars to be brought back.

In a sense we had all suffered brain damage at the time of Christopher's accident. This manifested itself in various ways: in particular, we would find our minds a total blank when we tried to remember specific names or precise words; even the names of familiar friends would be lost. How Guy managed to work, and Paddy and Hilary to study for their exams, I will never know. Shock stuns the brain, and recovery is a very slow process.

Things were in some ways easier for me. I had set myself a job to do which was so engrossing that it occupied me totally. I refused to think beyond the immediate moment and I had a strong belief that, if I worked with all my heart and strength, God would help me. I could not afford to doubt. As the months wore on, I began to realise more and more that it was essential for us all to behave in the manner which came naturally to us — more importantly, in a manner that *Chris* would recognise was in character. The mother's role in the family is that of caring, and attending to the more delicate functions of her child. The father and siblings have an altogether different relationship of sympathy, companionship and cheerful banter. It seemed important to me that this normal behaviour be preserved as far as possible. It was with this in mind that I decided to assume sole responsibility for all the nursing and attentions of personal hygiene that Chris would need once he was home. We agreed this and respected it over the years and I am convinced that this helped Chris to retain his dignity and take his place naturally amongst us despite his disabilities and dependence.

The design of the work I did for Chris only unfolded gradually; the direction was unclear in those early days, so I read everything to do with brain injury that I could lay my hands on. The eagerness with which I was prepared to explore any suggestion, however bizarre, was a measure of the desperation I felt at the paucity of information and help available. As a result of this attitude, I occasionally found myself in some unlikely places and strange situations. At one level I was alert to the humour of some of these actions, but at another I was determined to leave no stone unturned.

I remember one such occasion when a thoughtful friend told me of his concern that Chris had not been confirmed. Feeling that I should do nothing with which Chris might not agree if he was fully conscious, I declined his offer of help. But later that day, on the way to the hospital, I passed a Roman Catholic Church and decided to go in to pray, although I am not a Catholic. As I went in, I noticed a white enamel urn on a table by the door, bearing a roughly-written notice: 'HOLY WATER'. This arrangement seemed curiously comic and inappropriate to me, but on impulse, I emptied a flask I had with me and refilled it from the tap of the urn. Returning to the hospital, I made a cross on Christopher's forehead with the water. I felt sure that God would understand my tortured reasoning and accept my beloved Chris. I do not believe, and did not then think, that it would have mattered to God, but I suppose a sense of superstition prompted my action.

Some of the suggestions which were made to me I took up with considerable trepidation and diffidence. Often the help I obtained was of a very different kind from that which I had expected. One such case occurred when I was introduced to a remarkable faith healer, Mrs Winifred Durrant. This was something I would never have considered for one moment in the ordinary course of events, but as a result of my visit she wrote to me each week. Her letters brought release of the emotional tension which, despite my efforts to keep calm, would build up in my mind. It was a wonderful relief to be able to express my anxieties to someone who was totally sympathetic, yet not personally involved in our troubles.

But the stark fact of the matter remained: no person who had suffered the type and severity of brain injury that Christopher had sustained had ever been known to recover any useful mental function. I knew it was imperative, if he was to survive, that his mind be restored. Only then could he have the promise of a worthwhile life. His survival without a lively mind would be a living death. It is our mind which controls our personality and spirit: only through the mind is dignity, inspiration and usefulness given to our human existence.

Chapter Six

'All things work together for good'

It had been explained to me from the beginning that, whatever his condition, Chris would have to be transferred to another hospital at the end of nine months. I had been allowed such exceptional freedom in his handling at the Whittington Hospital that the thought of having to accept a transfer to a hospital where the authorities would be unlikely to show the same tolerance of my unorthodox methods was almost unbearable.

There was still almost everything to be done. By now I felt that Chris was aware of me and became relaxed in my presence, but I believed these delicate beginnings would be destroyed if I could not continue my work with the same insistence. It was necessary therefore to find the right hospital and another sympathetic consultant. This was a daunting task which would take up valuable time and effort. All my strength and energies were already being strained to the utmost. To have further demands made upon me of seeking, persuading and convincing strangers of the value of what I was doing, when already months of labour had shown no convincing results, seemed almost beyond me.

I felt intolerably weary, but nevertheless I began to contact the hospitals nearer our home to see if any of the medical staff would accept Chris. I was received sympathetically but, because the prognosis was so devastating and staff shortages acute, they declined. It was when this situation really dawned on me that I decided that, as soon as practicable, I would bring Chris home to be nursed. But in the meantime I had to continue my search for the best interim solution to the problem.

It had been my habit through these interminable months to visit the Reverend Phipps-Jones, a long-standing family friend who had always given support and comfort to us in our troubles. Now he advised me to approach Dr Christopher Woodard, a consultant psychiatrist and a man of strong faith, who might be able to recommend a colleague to me. This was arranged, but during our interview in his consulting rooms, I was dismayed to discover that, instead of the medical consultation I was expecting, our meeting was more of a mystical experience. Having listened to the medical and family history, he turned to prayer, full of an intense concentration. I had expected to receive concrete advice in the form of names and addresses and was desperately disappointed that at this eleventh hour I should apparently be wasting my time. No wonder he chided me about my lack of faith and my inability to let the Lord work his will! Feeling deeply dispirited, I said goodbye. He must have sensed my despair because he clasped both my hands and told me that the right person would be made known to me at the right time; that was God's will.

Wearily I retraced my steps to the hospital. Totally disheartened, I asked the doctor on duty to go ahead with whatever transfer arrangement he could make. Under the Health Service rules, after three months' stay in these specialised units, a patient had to be re-accepted by the hospital to which he had first been admitted. Immediately after his accident Chris had been taken by ambulance to the casualty department of Barnet General Hospital, but then sent straight on to the Whittington, where we had already been allowed an extra six months grace beyond the statutory period. I had not previously met the Registrar who happened to be on duty that day, but he was sympathetic and, realising how distressed I was, tried to console me. While he talked, my mind was elsewhere until I was suddenly made alert by his saying that he could probably arrange for his former boss, a consultant surgeon, to accept Chris. Out of politeness more than interest, I remember asking the surgeon's name.

As though in a dream I heard my strained voice say, 'Oh No — it can't be — I broke my engagement to him twenty five years ago, to marry my husband!'. The poor young Registrar (his first day on duty I learned later) fled horrified, so I was left alone to contemplate this scarcely extraordinary turn of events. I hope I will be forgiven by those concerned if I tell a little of this intimate story.

Guy and I are cousins: he is three months older than me; at the time of our dreadful dilemma over Chris we were both forty-nine years old, but when the Second World War had disrupted our lives we were nineteen years of age. We had known each other well all our lives, and had an affectionate relationship but it had nonetheless become central to my being that one day we should marry, though nothing was said of the matter by either of us. Once the war had absorbed us we followed quite different ways and scarcely saw one another for the next six years, hardly exchanging a letter.

During this time we naturally both experienced romantic relationships albeit never of a profound nature, but always I felt the restraint of my love for Guy: though undeclared it was nonetheless deeply felt. However, as the years went by, I met and developed a deep attachment to David, a medical student at my hospital, and I eventually became engaged to him. It was a provisional engagement: I told him of my love for someone of whose feelings for me I was uncertain and that only after he had found himself a wife elsewhere could our engagement become absolute.

This was the ambivalent state of my heart when, in 1945 the war in Europe ended and I found myself nursing at an army hospital in Egypt. Within a few months the war in Burma also ended. To my astonished delight, Guy reappeared as if from nowhere and, on the beach at Alexandria, I promised to marry him. So many years having been missed, we wasted no more of our lives and were married at Abassieh near Cairo as soon as formalities and the riot-stricken state of Egypt allowed this whirlwind change in our fortunes.

In due course I learned that my doctor friend had also married, had a family and had become a distinguished consultant surgeon. Now, in the very depth of my extremity, I heard his name being suggested as the person who might possibly accept Chris. Within a few minutes, this well nigh incredible coincidence was amazingly compounded, as I heard that the hospital where he worked was the Barnet General. This was the one hospital that was bound by National Health Service rules to take Christopher for indefinitely prolonged care. It was also the nearest and most convenient hospital to our home.

What was to be done in these new circumstances? I knew I had to write to tell David what had transpired, to give him the chance to refer my son's case to a colleague, if he so wished, although there was no one in the world to whom I could better trust his care. Once again Christopher's fate was put in the balance and we waited, helpless, for the outcome. David's response was positive and unhesitating and Christopher was transferred on 7th April, 1970. By the bedside of our stricken son, my husband and my ex-fiancé shook hands for the first time.

The only person *not* astonished by this outcome was Dr Woodard. The very afternoon following my consultation with him saw the end of my search. Since that time he has become a staunch and sympathetic friend, and it is as a result of his urging, now many years ago, that I have felt compelled to write this story.

Christopher was willingly accepted by my old friend as a patient and I was given every facility and freedom to work as I pleased. With my daily journey to the hospital now reduced to only about four miles, I had more time there. The staff were marvellous and welcoming, so that I felt immediately among friends. We were given a side room, so that when I was working with Chris I would not disturb the other patients. However,

David told me that this happy state of affairs could not be guaranteed beyond September (only four months away) as he was then due to take up a full-time appointment with a London teaching hospital and would have to leave Barnet. He obviously could not commit his successor to any arrangements which we had made: that would be entirely a matter for the new consultant.

My mind had been occupied for some time with plans to take Christopher home. If I was to follow my tentative timetable, this would happen about the end of August. I had chosen this date because it was a year from the accident and I felt it was long enough to be away from home. It seemed vital from the point of view of the rest of the family that we should all be together again and try to rebuild our family life. But I also believed that the earlier I could bring Chris home, the more likelihood there would be that our familiar surroundings would affect his re-awakening. Having explained this to my consultant friend, we agreed to work with that date as our goal. I had spoken of this as a possibility but certainly Guy and, I think, Patrick and Hilary, believed it was an unrealistic dream of mine.

As Chris showed only very slow improvement to me, and none at all to anybody else, I realised that if I kept to my proposed date, he would still be in a totally helpless state. He was still graded by the hospital as being in the most profound state of unconsciousness, though I myself felt that it was at a lighter level than when we had made the transfer. It was therefore important for me to consider and plan for every eventuality. He was of course still totally dependent for food and water on a naso-gastric tube permanently passed through his nose and down his throat, while his lungs required frequent suck-outs by means of a vacuum machine. Once he was home, although I could be supported and helped by others, control of the management of his condition would be my responsibility entirely and I knew that it would be a lonely and unrelieved task for many years.

Of all this I was keenly aware, but I also believed that it was the only way which offered any hope of a worthwhile quality of life for Chris. I felt he needed the constant inspiration of the familiar objects of home and family within the four walls of our own house to reassure him and to stimulate his mind, particularly while his conscious level was lightening.

All the time, while working with Chris at the hospital, I was mentally listing all the things needed for his homecoming. The first physical necessity was to arrange a downstairs room with easy access to the garden. The furniture had to be chosen with considerable care, since it not only had to be suitable for the purpose but easy to manage and attractive to look at; the room should be homely and pretty, but uncluttered. All the nursing and medical necessities had to be freely accessible and yet out of sight, so that the chilling atmosphere of a sick person's room could be done away with and visitors could feel welcome. This was particularly important because there is an almost instinctive fear, which everyone has to overcome, when faced with a situation so different and abnormal as Christopher's. So I put all the nursing utensils on a trolley which I covered with a pretty tablecloth and tucked it away in a corner of the room. It was then ready at a moment's notice to be pulled alongside his bed so that any procedures could be carried out quickly and efficiently.

I chose our dining room for him because its French windows opened onto a wide terrace from which friends later constructed a ramp into the garden. It was next to the kitchen, so I would always be within hearing distance and easy reach. Also, it was an attractive room, spacious, light and airy, at the same time its heavy curtains could darken the room entirely. This proved very beneficial as he quite frequently felt the need to have darkness and quiet; I think he sometimes suffered from a mild form of photophobia.

I sought everywhere for advice as to the best equipment and help available. From the Social Services I learned of the excellent facility of the Disabled Living Foundation headquarters.

There, on appointment, an occupational therapist will demonstrate a wide range of equipment for the handicapped. I found her tremendously helpful. While I was there she rang various firms to discover the availability of goods, current prices and delivery times. As a result of this visit I was able to suggest to the DHSS representative what items would be suitable for Chris. The bed, the hoist, commode and wheelchair were all provided free of charge, but other items we had to buy.

A hospital-type bed, a hoist and a wheelchair were the three items which had to be particularly carefully chosen. His bed needed to be versatile enough to enable me to carry out the various procedures of his exercise routine, regular postural drainage for his chest, frequent nursing attentions and constant changes of position. Sometimes he needed to lie flat, at other times to have the bed tipped, either at the foot or the head, and an adjustable back-rest was essential as an integral part of the frame. The bed I chose had all these variations easily controlled by a hand operated winching device; since speedy manipulation was important, this was ideal. There was a further advantage to this design, in that its height could be adjusted to enable particular procedures to be carried out at the most convenient level. This made things much easier for me, as I am not very tall and Chris was a full weight adult and totally helpless.

The hoist I chose was one of the pieces of equipment I most came to value. For the greater part of the time I was without help, so a hoist was essential for lifting Chris in and out of bed. There are a number of different types: some can be moved about the room on wheels, others can be attached to ceiling-rails. At first I used a mobile hoist because it could be moved discreetly out of the way when not in use, but later, when we moved to Gaterounds Farm, I had one attached to the ceiling because there was a bathroom adjoining his bedroom, and by then it was only needed for getting Chris in and out of the bath.

I had to consider the choice of wheelchair with equal care. They are in the main extremely uncomfortable, poorly designed and made with unsafe brakes. Fortunately, for several years before Chris' accident I had been a member of the Hertfordshire Association for the Welfare of the Handicapped. Working with disabled people, I had learned a good deal about the bad points of wheelchair design. I would advise anyone to ask a wheelchair user for their advice before committing themselves to a particular type — that is to say, someone who needs to use one day in, day out. Advisers at assessment centres are helpful but nothing can better experience gained from actual use. Most types of chair are available on prescription if the patient's GP recommends a particular design. One can either travel to a centre or an assessment officer will call. I have always found them helpful and full of ideas about how specific problems can be overcome.

Originally I used a fully reclining chair for Chris because for many years he could only sit up for short periods. This was fitted with adjustable leg supports as his circulation was so poor in those early days, and it was necessary to be able to raise his legs quickly so that the swelling which would develop when his feet were low could be quickly relieved.

I worked with a feverish intensity to get everything ready for Christopher's homecoming now that a moving day was set. All the time, while I was working with him at the hospital I noted the procedures and listed every need. They seemed almost endless; a vacuum suction machine was required to aspirate his lungs; a ripple mattress, to guard against pressure sores; all the complications that he might develop had to be anticipated, and equipment obtained that would be essential to deal with them. I listed the nursing equipment, bedpans and urinals, protective rubber sheeting and domestic appliances we would have to buy.

There were other items needed to help with the extra work involved in nursing Chris at home: a larger automatic washing machine, a food liquidiser, a new fire, and electric blanket to provide warmth over and above the fairly high background heating which is always required for persons who are paralysed. It is difficult to anticipate all that is needed in nursing a paralysed patient at home, the key is to be alert for sudden changes in their condition and to be able to take action immediately.

Nothing could be left to chance, because once I had him at home I knew I should have little opportunity of getting out to obtain anything that was lacking. Every contingency had to be catered for; Chris would be totally dependent on me, hour by hour for his very life. Most of the time I would be working single handed, unable to leave him even for short periods.

My status as an SRN was of considerable advantage in convincing people that I would be able to manage such a heavy nursing case at home. But none of the nursing procedures involved are beyond the capabilities of an intelligent, healthy and determined person. With a strong constitution, patience and a will to succeed, caring love will be rewarded beyond measure.

Chapter Seven

Homecoming

For some time, because Christopher's condition was apparently unchanging, we had felt that Guy's presence was needed more at home than at the hospital. Patrick and Hilary had been marvellous in their acceptance of Christopher's needs in the early weeks but, as time wore on, we felt that it was essential to attempt to make a more normal life for them.

It was now springtime; things always seem easier to cope with once winter is finished. With the spring and summer months ahead, I think we all felt a little better. Pressure for me was greatly eased with the move to the new hospital, as travelling times were considerably reduced.

During the four months following Christopher's admission to Barnet General Hospital, I felt that his unconscious state was slowly lightening. I believed he was aware of my presence, though I could see he was unresponsive to others; I believed too that his personality was reasserting itself. It was like watching the opening of a rose: first, the slightest loosening of the tight bud, then the tentative movement of one petal, then another.

The spring and summer were once again beautiful, and although Chris appeared totally unconscious to others I felt an impulsive need to get him away from the four walls of the hospital ward into the fresh air again. So each day, with the nurses' help to get him into a wheelchair, I would trundle him, well bolstered to keep him upright, onto the verandah or out into the hospital grounds.

One spring morning, after a gusty storm, I took him out as usual and discovered a fledgling sparrow, almost lifeless, at our feet. It had fallen from its ruined nest onto the ground. It was natural for me to pick it up and put it into Chris' hand. Immediately he cupped his hand and curled his fingers round it in a protective gesture. This would have been the instinctive response of the old Chris, and it was quite wonderful to witness. Of course the poor little thing died despite my best endeavours, but as a result of this, I asked if I could bring a guinea pig to the ward. I thought the soft warmth and life in it would touch a chord in his memory as he held it, being reminded of the guinea pigs he and the other two children had reared in Tanganyika.

At this time, believing that he could see in spite of what the doctors told me to the contrary, I brought our cine films of Africa to the hospital and projected them onto the white wall of his room. It appeared to me that his eyes, which normally would not be fixed on any particular object, would remain on the picture for quite a long time, as if it was somehow engaging his attention.

Gradually I became convinced that he knew me. One day, while returning him to his bed, I was suddenly overcome with a sense of loss. Without thinking I turned sadly to Chris and said, 'Of all the things lost, I most miss your smile. It will be so wonderful to see you smile again.' With a tremendous effort his face, which for so may months had been an expressionless mask, was transformed by a lop-sided grimace. It was a ghastly distorted smile, but it was all he could achieve and I knew that all the love, courage and hope of which his stout heart was capable was in it; the tears just coursed down my face. Over the next few weeks, he was able to produce this smile whenever he was asked. It really was the first sign that he acknowledged the presence of others.

It was towards the end of July 1970 that I first became aware of a subtle change in his condition. It seemed that the diurnal rhythm of waking by day and sleeping by night was now superimposed on his unconscious state. I had such a strong feeling that this was so that I felt unable to leave the hospital until he had relaxed into this state of so-called 'sleep' each night, usually at about 9.30pm. This of course meant that I was spending more and more time at the hospital, and reinforced my determination to bring him home as soon as it could possibly be managed.

It may seem that I was living in a state of unreality, altogether too calm for the circumstances, or that I am not able to recall the true picture of that time. Neither is right. I had to conserve my energies if I was going to succeed in the work I was trying to do for Chris; and not dissipate them by fruitless worrying. I forced myself to separate those matters that needed immediate attention and to put on one side what could be left for later consideration. This was almost a physical action. I had faith that when it became necessary to deal with them and I had the strength to cope, I could take them out again and an answer would be revealed. As for remembrance, these events have been burnt into my mind.

At this time then, I put into the back of my mind the last detail which still had to be settled before I could bring Chris home. This was that we would require the help of two people with very special qualities, one to help with our family and one to help with Chris. They should be experienced in nursing and be patient and tolerant, possessing both sympathy and a sense of humour. Above all, it was important that they should fit easily into our family life.

In the meantime, however, another pressing need had developed. It was now twelve months since the accident and the whole family had carried an almost intolerable burden of anxiety. It was essential to remove Patrick and Hilary for a while from this nightmare situation and, as far as was humanly possible, take them to a place out of communication with the world, particularly away from the distressing affairs at home. It was natural for our family to think in terms of mountains, and Guy decided that the Austrian Alps would best meet their needs. There they would be totally absorbed in intense activity, sleeping in mountain huts above the snow line, physically exhausted but mentally exhilarated. In these lovely surroundings I hoped they would be able to forge a philosophy which would help them to come to terms with our tragedy. This was arranged for the last fortnight in August and the first week in September, which fortuitously coincided with my tentative plan for Christopher's return home.

As the last arrangements for their holiday were being made, a telegram came out of the blue from my sister Rosemary in New Zealand. It was the answer to my prayer. Unasked, she had decided to take a year's leave from her job as an occupational therapist in Auckland Hospital to help with the family and Chris. Such extraordinary generosity I had not dreamt of, but here was the answer to one of the last problems needing solution before Chris could come home. Now I knew that the right moment had come and I could go ahead for a trial period. Rosemary, my sister, was the unique helper I was looking for. In the next three weeks, with the rest of the family away, she and I could give our undivided attention to bringing Chris home.

At this time too, I was contacted by Cathie Stroud, a nurse who lived locally and who, having heard about my plans, offered to come each morning to help me with the heavy nursing duties. She was absolutely lovely, and she became a dear friend: for five years, until we moved to our present home, we worked happily together.

And so I brought Chris home. Initially it had been decided by the hospital staff that he should just stay at home for two weeks, as a trial, but as soon he was safely tucked up in his own bed under our roof, I knew that I simply could not bear to send him back to the hospital. Come what may, I would have to manage, and a great load was lifted from my mind.

As every mother knows, from the moment her child is born and for as long as it is needed, she has accepted ultimate responsibility for another human being. This obligation places upon her shoulders a burden of work which, whatever measure of satisfaction it may give, is nevertheless endless. With me it was simply a matter of degree, and went beyond the age for which such care is usually necessary. It was in no spirit of martyrdom or arrogance that I undertook to nurse Chris at home, but simply because no other way that was offered held any hope of a worthwhile future for him.

Of course I realise that the consultant showed tremendous faith in my ability to cope by allowing Chris to come home in such a helpless condition. But professional qualifications such as I possessed are not a pre-requisite. Another family I know convinced their son's neurologist that they would be able to manage to nurse their son, and he was allowed home in a similarly dependent condition. They were not trained medically; they were farmers with a large and loving family and many good friends in their neighbourhood, all of whom were willing to assist. It *can* be done, but it takes its toll on the physical and mental resources of the family. However, I feel that it is in no way so great a strain as when the family is torn between attendance at the hospital and trying to sustain normality at home. It is certainly less stressful for the mother, but also, I believe, for the father and (if there are any) other children too. Out of sight does not mean out of mind; there is always a guilt feeling to be borne by the family at home.

At last I knew that I was free to work with Chris in circumstances where nothing would break the momentum or interfere with our programme. I know that if I had not brought him home at that time I would have regretted it for the rest of my life.

Over the next two weeks my sister and I established our routine. This was originally arranged as a fourteen day trial period while the family were away, after which Chris would be returned to the hospital. The idea was that, when the family had had time to assess the situation free from pressure, we would all determine whether to have Chris home permanently. I knew that this was a very sensible arrangement but, as the days went by, I realised there was no longer any possibility of turning back. He had settled so well and seemed altogether more relaxed. Now the rest of the family had to see this new state of affairs for themselves.

Having won the agreement of the consultant to this change of plan, I waited with growing nervousness for Guy, Patrick and Hilary to return from their mountaineering holiday. I know that it was a tremendous shock to them to discover the changes that had taken place in their absence. I am sure that their immediate inner response to finding Chris at home was one of dismay, and I am eternally grateful to them that they did not express such feelings. Many people felt that to take on such a serious and apparently quite hopeless case at home was to invite a breakdown in our family unity or of my health, and I'm sure that Guy particularly was fearful of this.

But, before long, they all felt that nothing could persuade them to send Chris back. Almost immediately we began to notice a perceptible improvement in his condition, although this would not have been detectable by anyone from outside. But there seemed to us to be a touching awakening, associated with pleasure at being home, that was encouraging to us all. However difficult the situation, we were determined to make it work now that we were all once more united as a family.

Chapter Eight

In Touch

After Chris returned home I knew it was important to preserve his self respect, independence and dignity in every way possible. His personality had to be allowed to develop. Never again would we have him as he had been amongst us, but the re-born Chris would be as though we had a third son, in some ways different but with essentially the same characteristics, loved for himself in his own right and not out of pity. I thought it was essential that we should each treat him in the same manner in which we had behaved to him in the past, and it was for this reason that I decided to carry out all the nursing duties and intimate attentions that he needed myself.

I know the rest of the family found this approach difficult. In many ways he had become a stranger to them. Visiting him in the hospital environment had somehow made him more remote, and his continued total unresponsiveness in any shape or form made it well nigh impossible to overcome this remoteness. Then, in November 1970, about three months after his return home, an event occurred that convinced them all that Chris was capable of an intelligent response.

When working with him, I constantly talked to him in a perfectly normal way, often in question form. On this particular occasion I had made some commonplace remark — 'Is that more comfy?' or some such thing — and I noticed a slight movement of the thumb of his right hand, just a slight extension. It was almost certainly a random uncontrolled muscular action — or was it? A tiny thrill touched my heart and with a scarcely controlled voice I dared to try again. 'Chris — Chris — are you sure you're comfy?' Without hesitation the thumb straightened up, even more strongly than before!

It is difficult for me to find words to convey to the reader who has had no such experience, what a giant leap forward this tiny gesture represented. One moment, my darling son was totally incapable of any form of communication: the next I had access for the first time in fifteen months to his precious mind. Until this time, I was the only person who suspected that his mental abilities had returned. For many months I had believed I could see intelligence in his eyes. Now, at last, he would be able to convince others.

All through the day I put questions to Chris, surprising him by the unexpected. My excitement mounted as I saw the quick responsive movement of his thumb. But, the nearer the hour drew to the time for Guy to come home, my nervousness increased. I knew so well the anxious look which would cloud his face as he approached Christopher's bedside, tormented and fearful as he was that I might allow my imagination and longing to build up false hope. I prayed with all my heart that Chris would respond to him. Through the months, Chris and I had built up a wordless communication, which was almost incredible to others, and now I was afraid this might prove to be just a further extension of our close understanding, still excluding others. How can I describe my anxiety of suppressed excitement as I told Guy of this wonderful development? When Guy went in to see Chris it seemed to me they should make this first communication alone; it seemed a holy moment.

The first sound I heard was the scraping of a chair as it was pulled close to Christopher's bedside. Then, after what seemed an endless period of silence, I heard Guy say, 'What is this, Chris?' following the question with a list of random names of mundane articles. As I peeped through the crack of the door, I saw Guy was holding up his black pocket comb. As soon as the word 'comb' was spoken, up went Christopher's thumb. I could sense Guy's disbelief; he could hardly bear to hope that this sign of Christopher's returning intelligence was real.

Then there followed a list of other objects, growing even more challenging, including simple sums and chemical names. At last Guy came out of the room, and for the first time since the accident had happened, I saw a dawning look of hope ignite his features. With this ability to communicate, the world could open up to Chris again and a new life made possible.

There was no doubt about it now. For the first time the whole family was convinced that Christopher still had a functioning mind inside his paralysed body, and now he had offered us a key to it. Day by day after this, communication improved, and what was more, with it his old sense of humour began to re-assert itself. This made caring for him so much easier, and in due course led to the expression of his ready wit which had always been such a delight.

Because of my constant attendance on Chris, I had always been aware of any change in his condition long before it was noticed by others, and I believe he was able to understand much of what was said and done considerably earlier than we could prove positively. I believe this may be the case with many brain-injured patients. There is the subconscious erection of a barrier between relatives and patient in any hospital ward, and without the existence of a communication channel, as had so far been the case with Chris, such a barrier can seem insurmountable. I think there is a strong possibility that distress could be caused by well meaning attendants inadvertently discussing the condition of an 'unconscious' — that is to say, totally unresponsive — patient, within his or her hearing. Years later, in the Intensive Therapy Unit of the Royal Free Hospital, I was delighted to see on the wall behind each patient's bed, a notice saying 'PLEASE REMEMBER ALL OUR PATIENTS CAN HEAR'. I believe that this was so in Christopher's case, as he subsequently showed a marked antipathy towards anyone he considered to be associated with hospitals.

On one occasion my sister, who had by then taken a part-time post as an occupational therapist in a local hospital, returned home still wearing her uniform. As she approached his bed he became distraught and only calmed down when she changed her clothes and he realised who she was. Normally he recognised her without difficulty and loved to have her help him, but his behaviour on this occasion was quite unexpected and out of character. Likewise he would become very agitated and unco-operative when doctors tried to examine him. These examinations later became necessary because we had a legal case pending relating to the accident and, in order to win his co-operation, we had to introduce them as friends of the family who were simply interested in seeing how much improvement he was making.

After he came home I kept a record detailing Christopher's physical, emotional and mental condition, at first making assessments at six monthly intervals, later shortened to two months when the rate of change increased. The improvement in his condition was exceedingly slow, but it was steadily progressive. I can remember feeling desperately lonely at times and uncertain that what I was doing was the right thing for Chris and the family, but a retrospective study of his progress as revealed in my notebook reassured and encouraged me.

As he was still utterly helpless, I was not able to leave him alone for more than a few minutes at a time, so I slept on a couch in his room for the first eighteen months. This was also necessary because he required two hourly nursing attention, day and night: naso-gastric feeds had to be given, pressure points massaged, his chest cleared and so on.

Thankfully, in the spring of 1971, eight months after I had brought him home, I was able to dispense with the naso-gastric feeding. He was becoming increasingly distressed by the nasal tube; I think that the returning sensitivity of his pharynx must have made it intolerable. Although his swallowing reflex was slow to return and unreliable at first, with patience I was able to give him some food by mouth; but he was not able to manage thin fluids without paroxysms of choking for another four years. It was yoghurt that proved to be the perfect medium, and I liquidised this with puréed protein, fruit, vegetables and other things.

Over the years I have used gallons and gallons of yoghurt — usually the plain natural kind, but Chris also loved the fruit flavoured varieties. Yoghurt had the particular quality of not breaking up in the mouth in the way that custard or cornflour can, nor melting like ice-cream or jelly. However, for about a month after I started this transition, he was simply not able to take in enough liquid by mouth, so once a day I had to re-pass the wretched naso-gastric tube — a perfectly beastly job, because he objected to it more and more.

Towards the end, the only way I could succeed was to pass it after he was asleep at night. During this period I gave him two-hourly feeds of twice the usual volume throughout the night while he slept, to keep his fluid balance correct, only gradually decreasing this as his ability to swallow improved. All in all, it was a difficult and slow process, but very very gradually his swallowing improved and I was able to coarsen the texture of his food until after nearly ten years he was eventually weaned onto a normal diet.

Although in the early years he suffered some emotional disturbances, I was adamant that he should not be given tranquillisers. I felt that it was of vital importance that nothing should be given that might cloud his mind. It was always possible to calm and comfort him with soft endearments and gentle caresses in exactly the same way that one would soothe a troubled child. Indeed, for the first few years following his accident I felt that, without being able to explain why, he was emotionally dependent on me just as he had been when he was a baby. Later when his communicative abilities developed, I discovered that the intellectual and emotional sides of his personality were working at different levels, as though they were split. The intellectual side of his brain returned at its adult level, but the emotional side of his brain recovered through similar phases and in the same order as it had developed through childhood, though in a much-reduced time-scale. Eventually the two sides came together and his mental state became mature and stable.

Partly out of habit from my nursing days, but also because I knew that I was witnessing a profoundly interesting recovery, I kept meticulous records of Christopher's treatment and observation of his condition for many years. I wrote everything down, each procedure was timed and recorded, and I disciplined myself to keep to his timetable, however tired I felt: I simply forced myself to get on with the work.

By the summer of 1971 my sister Rosemary had to return to New Zealand. Her help through that first year of nursing Chris at home had been invaluable. She was irreplaceable, and we all sadly missed her lovely warm personality. I could not imagine how I would manage without her, but fortunately Cathie Stroud, the nurse who had already been helping me with Chris, was able to come each day to give a hand. She became a family friend and a firm favourite with Chris. Her wonderful air of cheerfulness and her ability to tackle any job with vigour and humour won our hearts. She was always totally dependable, and I know that I could never have managed those early years without her help.

All through the years the most remarkable fact about Christopher's recovery was its steady progress. Although we were thankful to see his physical improvement, it was the change in his mental condition which was most gratifying. The fleeting moments of awareness, which I had first noticed about eleven months after his accident, gradually lengthened and the troughs of withdrawal became shallower until his condition became the normal conscious state of wakefulness by day and sleep by night.

About three months after he came home we were able to test Christopher's memory and intelligence by putting a question to him and asking him to raise his thumb for the correct answer, which we had put amongst a list of false ones. His memory of specific subjects from his academic work and general knowledge was very good. His thumb movement was slight but immediate and we could sense his delight at this new found ability to release his thoughts. In this way we were able to discover that his memory of events was clear up to two years before his accident: to be precise, the latest date he was able to recall was 24th June 1967.

Quite early on he developed a unique method of finger writing across his chest with his right hand, using 'mirror' writing so that anyone standing in front of him could understand its meaning. He invented this entirely of his own accord, and it enabled him to express himself, his thoughts and wants. It must have been a wonderful release to him.

At this time too it was clear that his hearing was fully restored and very acute. I believe that he could hear what was said much earlier than could be demonstrated practically, and I think he had probably understood what I was saying even when I had been working with him in hospital in the early days. I also discovered that his sense of smell had fully returned, and later when he was taking food by mouth, his sense of taste was found to be equally keen.

All the while he had been unconscious Christopher's eyes had been staring and empty of meaning. He blinked aimlessly — not in response to any particular stimulus, but at least sufficiently to keep his eyes in good health. As his sleep rhythm developed, he would close them at night. He had a nystagmus, that is, an unco-ordinated oscillation of the eyeballs, his left eye being more slow to move and its pupil failing to respond so well to light as his right eye did. However, as his consciousness returned I soon realised that he had useful vision; the realisation that he recognised me — to see the look of recognition in his face and the smile that went with it — was one of the most rewarding and heart-warming moments of my life.

It was soon clear that he recognised us all, family and friends, and in this way his quality of life was already enormously enhanced. He was not able to read normal-sized print for a number of years, but reading large sized script, just a few words at a time, was possible even from these early days. Gradually his eye movement improved, the nystagmus subsided, reducing the double vision that he almost certainly suffered, at least when he was tired. Though he was never again able to read a page of close-set type, he was able eventually to read well spaced uncluttered lines such as one finds in poetry books or captions to illustrations. Thus he regained his pleasure in looking at our various books on art and natural history, or using a globe to pick out countries and place names mentioned on the radio.

Coming as we did from a land in which there had been no television, we had been highly critical, contemptuous even, of the obvious deficiencies of much of what is presented on British television. But what a blessing it was to become for Chris, and how thankful we were that he had been spared sufficient sight to enable him to enjoy it.

From the earliest days of his recovery his quick wit was apparent. He was always as ready to prick pomposity as to show sympathy. There was a curious circumstance which indicated to me that, if a message was given with sufficient insistence and frequently enough, it was stored in his memory long before we had been able to recognise that his ability to memorise had returned.

At the time of the Watergate affair in the USA, the hearings of which began on 17th May 1973, none of us believed that Christopher was capable of taking a deep interest in external events. However, it was my habit to leave the radio on in his room as a stimulus to break the monotony of his day. Unfortunately our programmes were constantly filled with references to Richard Nixon and Watergate. For several years afterwards, Chris developed an obsession about the matter. In moments of emotional disturbance, or if he was not well, he would become distressed at any allusion to the subject, even confusing his everyday experiences and close family ties with it as though he was living in a bad dream. This anxiety was of such a degree that I had to distract him and turn off the radio at the slightest mention of the subject. As all the media seemed equally obsessed with the topic, this made things very difficult, forcing me to resort to the use of a tape recorder. Fortunately, as his mental condition returned to normal, so thankfully did the BBC!

He suffered another delusion which persisted for some years. When we moved to Gaterounds Farm in 1975, he believed that we had moved to New Zealand. We had spent the whole of 1957 there during his childhood and this had made a deep impression on him. I think he attempted to rationalise the situation of our move by imagining that we had returned there to be amongst my own family. His impression was undoubtedly strengthened by the fact that both my twin sister Ray, and Rosemary were visiting us from New Zealand at that time too. This was Rosemary's second trip to help me with Christopher's nursing, and it was to last four years, Our house seemed to be constantly full of New Zealand visitors. Once again, it seemed that an impression was being repeatedly reinforced upon his consciousness until it became a belief.

He would sometimes ask me what had happened between that precise date of 24th June 1967 to the present time. The gap caused him some distress and whenever he was tired or unwell the problem of the date would agitate him; because of this, I made sure that he always had a large clear calendar close at hand for reassurance. Gradually, as the years passed, I noticed that the time gap between 1967 and the date of his accident, 1969, was closing, and latterly he was able to recall events within eight months of that terrible time. But when he tried to account for the period of his unconsciousness he would become anxious; gently I would explain what had happened, and he eventually came to accept this.

At each stage the improvements in Christopher's condition

were only tentative, too slight to be noticed by anyone but me. I think a mother is always the first to notice change in a child's condition. It was like this when Christopher's speech began to return. At first I picked up his words by placing a stethoscope against his throat, but gradually the vocal chords strengthened. So much muscular effort is needed for speech; there are the muscles of the throat, tongue and lips, as well as those for breath control, of the chest and the diaphragm.

One difficulty he did not have was the choosing of the right words; his speech was difficult to follow in the early years because of muscular weakness and poor co-ordination of the physical control, not because of any mental block. But gradually it strengthened, as all his muscular actions did, and he was able to converse once more. This was a tremendously important step because it did away with the constant need for my mediation. Speech, after all, is the earliest communicative skill that any of us learns.

Chapter Nine

Out and About

Through the next few years our lives continued with very little change. Guy's work base had been transferred to Surrey at the time of Christopher's homecoming, which meant that he had to commute weekly to Hertfordshire. He would arrive home weary and dispirited each Friday evening, to return to work on Sunday evening. For him these were years of searing loneliness: he was consumed with anxiety throughout the week, and when he came home he felt helpless.

My life, in some ways, was easier by comparison: I knew what I had to do and was too busy to think. I just had to put my head down and get on with the job of looking after Chris, Patrick and Hilary. The strict routine of work which I had been forced to establish was something that it was difficult for Guy to become involved in, but of course his presence and involvement with Patrick and Hilary were vital.

Despite the grey dreariness of those years there were family achievements which were a source of quiet pride. When such a devastating blow strikes a united and loving family, the survivors become highly sensitised. It becomes important that somehow they should be seen, not to be bowed down by the adversity, but standing tall and flying a flag in defiance of it.

W.E. Henley expressed it so well:

> *In the fell clutch of circumstance*
> *I have not winced nor cried aloud:*
> *Under the bludgeonings of chance*
> *My head is bloody, but unbowed.*

Patrick had followed in his brother's footsteps to Buckingham Palace to receive the Duke of Edinburgh's Gold Award. Neither Guy nor I felt that we could go alone with him with such aching memories of Christopher's great day in our minds, and yet we dearly wished to share his proud moment. Unbeknown to me, Guy had written to the Award Scheme Secretary, telling him of our bitter dilemma. Within a few days, he received a special dispensation for both of us to attend, together with a car pass to permit us to drive into the inner courtyard of Buckingham Palace through the main gates — something it is nice to have done once in a lifetime!

We received later a parcel from the Palace containing Paul Bates' book, *The Horizontal Man* accompanied by a kind letter from the Duke's Personal Secretary, saying that it was sent at the express wish of Prince Philip to encourage Chris in his struggle to achieve a worthwhile life. We will never forget this kindness, which was so valuable to our family morale at a time of near despair.

Unfortunately, Hilary's school did not participate in the Duke of Edinburgh's award scheme at that time. In normal circumstances it would have been something she would have loved to tackle, a challenge which would have been met with ability and enthusiasm. Learning to drive, an accomplishment which is generally undertaken in late teens with the family backing, was also denied her due to our peculiar circumstances at that time. However, there was one love that she was able to pursue, which has remained a king-pin in her life, and that was horse-riding. She became a proficient horsewoman and has managed and kept horses in both England and Canada, in the latter building up her own riding school when she lived in Nova Scotia.

Patrick and Hilary, in spite of their stressed home base, succeeded wonderfully with their 'O' and 'A' level examinations, and both achieved university entrance. As a result of constantly visiting his brother in hospital, Paddy's thoughts had crystallised into a desire to study medicine, and it was at this time he began his medical studies at the Middlesex Hospital in London. Meanwhile, Hilary was accepted for a degree course in Horticultural Science at Reading University.

From the beginning, Guy and I had determined that, as far as it lay in our power, we would not allow Christopher's accident to spoil their lives. Annual family holidays were no longer possible, but Guy organised several challenging adventures with Hilary and Paddy. They climbed in Austria and the Swiss Alps, and on one notable morning, Paddy and Guy reached the summit of the Matterhorn.

Chris and I were only able to enjoy these trips vicariously, and I felt increasingly that we should try to break down the barriers of isolation for Chris too. For this we would need specialised transport. He was still totally helpless — a tetraplegic, paralysed in arms and legs, unable to move his head or speak properly. Any vehicle we chose would need easy access, good height, and space so that we could attend to him while we were travelling.

Knowing nothing about large vehicles, we decided to visit the Commercial Exhibition at Olympia. There someone told us that local county councils would sometimes sell used ambulances for the use of disabled people. Eventually we obtained a 30cwt Commer ambulance with a rear hydraulic lift, from a voluntary society in Hertfordshire. With expert and concerned assistance from a special unit at Rootes Motors, this was converted into the perfect vehicle for Christopher's particular needs.

Most of the seats were removed to provide space for a bed and to give a clear working area. The bed was mounted on heavy duty springs to reduce vibration, and fitted with safety belts and adjustable back-rest. A sprung platform was provided, to which his wheelchair could be anchored. To ensure adequate warmth, which was vital because his circulation was still poor, we had the van curtained and carpeted, and I always carried a 'space blanket' to provide ready warmth in an emergency.

Storage space was available under the bed, to stow equipment so that we had clear access to Chris at all times.

In case we should get into trouble while travelling with him, our vehicle was painted a bright daffodil yellow so that it could be easily identified. We called it 'Dobbin' and thus began our association with this friendly vehicle by means of which the world was once more opened up for Chris.

Our journeys began the day Dobbin was delivered to us. We decided to test its usefulness by taking a picnic to the nearby woods. It was a lovely autumn day, the sun was shining and the colours beautiful, and for the first time in three years we were able to introduce Chris again to the natural life he had loved so much. It was thrilling to watch his response. We boiled a kettle on a wood fire and brought fruits and leaves for him to identify. It was one of the most rewarding days with the family that I can remember. During the spring and summer of the following year we were able to be more daring in our outings and Dobbin proved to be everything we had hoped for.

A particular opportunity afforded to us with Dobbin was that we were able to take up an invitation which helped me tremendously with the problem of exercising Christopher's limbs. At that time, in the early 1970s, no hydrotherapy or domiciliary physiotherapy was available to the disabled housebound. Resources were limited and Christopher's condition so unusually dependent that, even today in similar circumstances, I doubt if they would be provided.

Some years later when we first went to Surrey, I was offered the services of a physiotherapist, through a system whereby we made voluntary contributions to the Society that employed her. She visited once a week for half an hour, over a period of three months, but at the end of this time she admitted that so little progress had been made that there was no point in continuing.

This was no surprise to me; I had only gone along with the idea because I did not want to seem to reject any help offered. She had insisted on working on her own, preferring to be alone with her patient. I knew how slowly any physical change in Christopher's condition came about, and I also felt it was a waste of her time; she would have been much better employed helping people over short term difficulties. But it did seem to me that her help might have been better used to train the patient's relatives in the procedures, which they could then carry out regularly and frequently. Her weekly visit could then have been of a supervisory nature. Over the years I had learned how important it was to make any message to the brain insistent and regular.

But now help came from an unexpected quarter. A friend gave me a press cutting about a man who was making exercising bikes for spastic children to strengthen their limbs and so help them towards their goal of walking. He worked from his own home in east London, and had little help from officialdom, although a church hall was made available to him, where the children and their mothers could work with his bikes. Small voluntary contributions were made towards his work, but he was mainly dependent on a supply of old discarded bicycles. We had two such bikes so, having arranged a visit, Chris and I set off in Dobbin on the first fine day.

It was an extraordinary experience. I felt I had met a kindred spirit: someone driven by a dream, dedicated to working towards a goal that few had faith in. He was a Napoleon of the back streets; his shed and kitchen were full of old bicycle frames in various stages of dismemberment. He made his devices by welding two front halves of bicycles together so that the pedals and their cogs could be driven by a common chain connected vertically. It was made stable by two sets of handlebars welded to the lower frame. The upper pedals were replaced by hand grips. This extraordinary contraption was then attached to the wheelchair in which the child was sitting. With both feet on the pedals, and hands on the grips, the chain would be slowly turned, according to the strength of the child's legs and arms.

I was witness to the success of his methods when I visited the church hall and listened to the mother's accounts of the way their children had improved. Above all I was impressed by the hope that was given them — a practical step to help their children when all had seemed lost.

Some days later, my Napoleon of the East End turned up at our house with Christopher's machine. It was a strange contraption indeed, and for the first year or two I found that I had to secure Christopher's hands and feet to it, until he grew stronger. To start with, he was dependent on me to push the pedals for him. But as time went by, he was able to drive the whole thing by himself, using his stronger right side to force movement upon his left.

Many brain-injured subjects develop flexion contractures of the knee and hips. I don't know why this was not a complication in Christopher's case. Perhaps it was in part due to the movements of his limbs that I forced upon him whenever his condition allowed, from the earliest days, and despite his total helplessness. Whatever the reason, we were lucky, because these distortions are difficult to correct.

Hilary and I travelled with Chris to the Cambridgeshire Fens to stay with a friend in her cottage. This gave us experience in the management of Chris away from home. Later we hired a caravan which we towed behind Dobbin and Guy and I took Chris to Suffolk and the Cotswolds. We went to the Constable country thinking it might revive his interest in painting, and while we were there we were involved in one of the typical mishaps that can overtake anyone travelling with a helpless person.

Knowing that one of the earliest paintings by Constable could be found in a church at East Bergholt, we decided to take Chris to see it, although I had not realised that we would have to take him up the altar steps if we were to get a close view. At this time we were not very experienced in the management of wheelchairs, and after some pushing and shoving, poor Chris was tipped out! He didn't hurt himself, but it took us a long time to restore the situation, such was our state of consternation mixed with hysterical laughter. We shan't easily forget where that particular painting can be found.

It was on our visit to the Cotswolds that I was able to realise a long cherished wish. Earlier that year, in March 1974, publicity had been given to the court case that we had contested for compensation for Chris. The circumstances of my nursing him at home had been publicised and as a result I had been contacted by the parents of a brain-injured boy who lived in Wiltshire. We had corresponded and spoken on the phone, but on this visit I was able to meet them and see for myself how they were coping with their son.

Doreen and Tom Slattery owned a farm and had a joyous family of ten children. Immediately Chris and I were welcomed as long-standing friends, and given an invitation to stay on the farm as often as we could. This was marvellous because I was able to watch Christopher's warm response to them and their family — his first real social contact with strangers since he had recovered consciousness. They had a small mixed livestock farm and Chris was able to share in the various activities. His excitement at sitting among young piglets and watching the hens being fed and the cows milked was clear to see. He loved it all and our ideas that any financial compensation for his accident should be used to provide him with a farming environment in the future were confirmed by this experience. From then on we began a search for a suitable small-holding within reach of Guy's work in Surrey.

We now had to turn our thoughts to the legal side of Christopher's accident. We had known all along that there were virtually no witnesses on that fateful evening, and what information we had been able to glean about the accident was slight. It seemed that it was the result of a momentary lack of concentration by the driver of a mini van, who was taking his girlfriend out for the evening. They were out of cigarettes and so were cruising quite slowly along the apparently clear high street looking for a tobacconist's shop. Chris was coming up behind them and pulled out to overtake just as the driver, having seen a shop still open, veered across the road in front of him. Chris, of whom he was totally unaware, apparently went into a skid trying to avoid the van, and spun off the road headlong into a brick wall.

Thus it was that this glorious young life was sacrificed for a cigarette. Despite wearing the best type of crash helmet available at that time, he suffered brain stem damage resulting in the devastating condition that I have described. So now we had to address the question of seeking financial help to secure the best possible future for him.

The insurance company of the other vehicle involved in the accident had offered only totally inadequate compensation to Chris, and it was therefore necessary to have recourse to the courts, if anything approaching justice was to be done. This was something that we approached with the utmost reluctance. Fortunately we had a wonderful family friend, John Talbot, a solicitor, who worked untiringly on our behalf. From the first days after the accident he had calmly stepped in and set in motion all the proper processes, and since Christopher himself had no financial resources, John was able to obtain legal aid for him.

This was also a practical contribution Guy could make on Christopher's behalf, and together John and Guy threw themselves into the task of gathering evidence and developing arguments that could convince Counsel to represent us in the High Court. This was an agonising experience for Guy: not only did it repeatedly stir old memories, but he had an innate antipathy to anything to do with litigation. But it was a vital part of working towards a worthwhile future for Chris.

We were not asking for compensation for what had been lost; how could anyone begin to assess that in material terms? But we did need financial help to provide a new way of life for Chris. This would need to be one in which his talents and interests could once more be engaged, and we had begun to believe that a small farming enterprise would offer such an opportunity.

The major difficulty which had to be overcome was to persuade a judge that the expectation of life for Chris was reasonably normal for his age, despite his medical history, for it is predominantly on this consideration that compensation is assessed by the insurance companies. Consistently the most hopeless prognoses had been presented to them by their neurological consultants who examined Chris. We could understand their dilemma, but we believed that they were biased by their experience of previous case histories and that they were misjudging Christopher's condition. They were strangers to Chris and our family and were unable to recognise his incipient strength, his determination and returning mental abilities. With every year that passed, his expectation of life was extended rather than decreased. The suggested periods of probable survival were consistently trailing reality, always having to be revised upwards. Far from being impatient with the law's delays, we knew that time (and, indeed, inflation!) were on our side.

Eventually on 4th March 1974, over four and a half years after the accident, our case came to the High Court in London before Mr Justice Brabin and agreed judgement was given in favour of Chris for the sum of £30,000. Much higher awards are of course becoming frequent, but liability was disputed and even at that time, we were up against opinion that he would only survive for a few years. However, this sum was sufficient, when combined with our only other financial resource — the sale price of our Hertfordshire house — to buy a tiny farm of twenty one acres in Surrey. The farmhouse had a self-contained ground floor extension which provided ideal accommodation for Chris.

So Gaterounds Farm was purchased and our new life began.

Chapter Ten

A Village Affair

We had considered long and hard before making up our minds to accept the challenge of this new way of life. Guy is a veterinary surgeon, and therefore qualified in animal husbandry, as well as in all the branches of veterinary medicine and surgery. So we felt well equipped to tackle the farming side of the enterprise, which we built up slowly from one cow, a horse, a sheepdog and a few hens. We expanded our stock as we felt able to take on more work.

Guy was working as a researcher in veterinary therapeutics; this meant that he was the adviser and I the farm labourer, though he was able to help with the physical work at weekends. Our first cow was a lovely in-calf Jersey. She had sustained an injury to her hip at birth which meant that she was at risk while running with the rest of the pedigree herd. Her owner, having been told by mutual friends of our plans, gave Lyric to us as a gift. She became our house cow and I became the milkmaid. I had a three-legged stool, and with my head resting against her flanks, I learned the gentle and beautiful art of milking. The soft, contented sound of her munching, the low rumble of her stomach and the peace of the stable was a wonderful therapy. I can recommend it to anyone under pressure — it is more effective than any psychiatrist's couch.

However we knew that it would be the emotional problems resulting from uprooting Chris which we might find more difficult. Although he had become used to visiting new places, he always returned home thankfully. I felt this was akin to the home-longing of Mole, described so sensitively in Kenneth

Grahame's *The Wind in the Willows*. Chris felt safe at Birch, our old home, and now we were proposing to loose his hold on this secure base, something which might well confuse and disorientate him. But however difficult the settling in might be, we felt we had to accept the risks because of the opportunities the move presented. It seemed to us to be a culmination of all we had been able to do so far for Chris.

The first major hurdle to be overcome was to sell our house. To facilitate this I felt it was important to keep any signs of an invalid-in-residence as unobtrusive as possible. Therefore every time anyone wished to view, I would put Chris in an old shirt and set him in front of a canvas on my easel, in a studio extension of the house. In this way he passed off as an eccentric artist friend at work, and no one felt they should intrude on his privacy. Meanwhile I polished and prettied the house, filling it with bowls of fragrant hyacinths, while Guy tidied the garden. Within four months the house was sold and in April 1975 we moved to Gaterounds Farm. Moving house with Chris while he was still in need of such complete nursing care was difficult, but I put everything he would need into Dobbin and dealt with the move as though we were going away on a holiday.

Patrick and Hilary — away at university — were thrilled with our new home and tremendously supportive of our plans. For one thing it meant that Hilary could at last buy her own horse, a beautiful Welsh cob, called Trojan. We rented out two of our stables to local horse-owners who were able to look after Trojan and exercise him while Hilary was away; that was happily arranged as part payment of the rent.

To help Chris settle in to the new surroundings I tried to make his new room look as much like the old one as possible. His ornaments, furniture and pictures were arranged as nearly as possible to their old position in relation to his bed. Even though I took pains to reassure him, he did suffer periods of confusion and withdrawal after the move. But after a time it was only when he was ill or tired that we saw any relapse into those disturbed states. The move proved to be a tremendous success and opened up a positive approach to the future for us all. We would not have decided to make the move for any other reason than that it would be helpful to Chris, but it also provided us, as a family, with a definite psychological break with the past and its sad memories.

For the first year at Gaterounds we were fully engaged in coming to terms with our new way of life. The happiest immediate result of the move was that Guy was able to travel from home to his laboratory each day, but once he returned at night we were always busy. Our new home was a sixteenth century traditional timber-framed farmhouse: like the Forth Bridge, it required constant care and maintenance, but we could not grudge the work, considering it a privilege to own such a beautiful place.

We wanted to start our livestock enterprise as soon as possible, so when the spring grass came we went to market and bought a dozen young heifers, so that we could begin rearing Hereford beef calves. Of necessity, through the day the care of these animals fell to me. Added to this were the household chores and the full time nursing which Chris still required. Every moment of our waking day was taken up with the work and we badly needed help.

Once again my sister Rosemary came to our aid. None of us guessed that this time it would mean a stay of nearly four years before she returned to New Zealand. Her understanding, sympathy and keen sense of humour put colour and fun back into all our lives once more. Rosemary's was a delightfully unpredictable character that could sometimes be thought to verge on eccentricity — unfairly perhaps, because there was usually a strange rationality behind such incidents. Perhaps an example will suffice to illustrate.

In moving to Gaterounds we had changed our local health authority and Christopher had to be re-assessed for all his special equipment, including a new wheelchair. In confirming the

Wheelchair Assessor's visit I had mentioned that if there was no response to the front doorbell, he should walk over to the farmyard, as I might be there with Chris working with our cows. It did not occur to me to mention his visit to my sister.

Rosemary had chosen this particular day to bleach her hair, using a product that, curiously, was coloured a vivid bilious green. After applying the material liberally she had then sealed her hair up in a gaudy plastic bag from a local supermarket. Combined with a long sweeping purple skirt, her ensemble was at the least bizarre!

Busy in the house, I failed to hear the official's ring: and he proceeded, as arranged, to the farm yard. Rosemary, occupied with her new vocational pursuit of rabbit keeping, heard footsteps that she took to be mine. But at the last moment, realising that a stranger was approaching, took fright and tried to hide at the back of a cow stall. He, however, had caught sight of a disappearing bit of purple skirt and assuming that the person he sought was wearing it, followed her in and confronted her.

Only afterwards did Rosemary realise that the green substance had been running down her face in sticky streaks making her look like something from a horror video. Speechless, she stood and pointed to the house, but the petrified young man was having none of it — white and shaken he turned and bolted to his car! He was about to make his escape when I, quite ignorant of what had happened, chanced to see him and call him back.

A true professional, he made no mention of the monstrous apparition he had met in the cowshed. We concluded the business of Chris' wheelchair without any further trouble, but I never saw him again. I imagine he dined out for some time on that tale of a 'Day in the Life of a Wheelchair Assessor'!

This hilarious experience was so typical of Rosemary's gloriously eccentric approach to life which, to her nephews and nieces, was a source of continual delight. There are far too few aunts of her calibre to keep the world sane today: I think perhaps our family's Irish connection must somehow have surfaced in her. Whatever it was, all children loved and treasured her.

As Rosemary was a trained occupational therapist her help and advice with Chris' exercises were invaluable. Even so, during this year, 1975, I became increasingly aware that I was reaching a point beyond which I could make no further progress. I simply did not know, and no one could tell me, how to advance a totally prone patient to a condition where he could stand upright and so make walking a real possibility.

It was soon after this, in August 1976, that I was given a book written by an American physiotherapist, Glen Doman. *What to do about your Brain-injured Child* described how it was possible to restore mental function and physical abilities to brain injured children by the stimulation of the senses and an insistent regimen of 'patterning'. These are exercises which have been devised to copy as nearly as possible those actions which are natural to a normal child progressing from birth to walking. Although the work which Glen Doman described was related entirely to young children, I felt I would be able to adapt the exercises to suit Christopher. I wrote to ask the British Institute of Human Potential if they were able to accept Chris as a patient, but they replied that they likewise only accepted children.

In retrospect I think this was just as well because after such a long time of working independently with Chris, I would have found it very difficult to relinquish control to others. I just was grateful that I now had a way to follow. So I set about making my own programme, using Glen Doman's book as a guide. In this way I was able to extract whatever I felt would be helpful to Chris and disregard everything irrelevant. This would have been impossible if I had not kept to myself the sole responsibility for his management.

To succeed I needed the help of some sixty volunteers each week. They had to work in teams of five, morning and evening, and be prepared to carry out the programme with vigour and perseverance probably for years. At this time, as can be imagined, we had not had any opportunity to make local friendships as we were so preoccupied at home. Curiously, one of the criteria we had listed as important when we were house hunting was that we should be within walking distance of a village. We were anxious to become part of a community, but at the time I had no idea what a vital piece in the jigsaw of Christopher's recovery this was to be. Now that I had to 'go out into the highways and byways' to gather helpers, I was thankful we were not isolated.

Our general practitioner, Dr Russell, was sympathetic to the idea and wrote a letter in our parish newsletter asking for volunteers. Although we had a good response from this source, many more were needed. So I decided to ask anyone who was thrown in my path to help. The day after I had finished Glen Doman's book, I was gazing out of the kitchen window when I noticed an Aberdeen Angus bull disporting himself amongst our heifers. As Guy was away, I had to ask its owner, our farming neighbour, to drive him back to his own field. As we were walking up the field with Englebert the bull in shamefaced retreat, I asked this perfect stranger if he would help me with the exercises. He was taken aback but being at something of a disadvantage gave in gracefully, promising not only his own help but that of his wife and family as well. Since that day they have proved staunch friends and were instrumental in recruiting many other helpers who gave unstinting help for over seven years.

Soon our list was full and I had made out a rota. We prepared an exercising pallet which we could lay on top of Christopher's bed and I equipped him with suitable protective clothing. For this, track suits were ideal because, as well as being trim and easily washed, they made him look like any other young man of his age about to take up athletics. By September 1976, after a month of intensive preparation, we were ready to begin.

As a result of these twice-daily sessions of exercises and stimulation, we succeeded in restoring Chris to a condition I had hardly dared hope for. When we started the exercises Chris bitterly resented this interference by strangers and this resulted in outbursts of unco-operative behaviour. I sometimes felt so ashamed of these struggles that I almost discontinued the exercises, feeling that I should not subject my helpers to this. However, they were made of sterner stuff than I had given them credit for and battled through until the stormy scenes gave way to willing co-operation.

It was not long before Chris was making the most of these social occasions. There was usually one Delilah in the team, more tolerant than the others, who would allow Chris to flirt outrageously with her. He had always had an eye for a pretty girl. Altogether he was much indulged and it added an entirely new dimension to his life. We had gloriously happy times with laughter ringing through the house. Our conversation ranged through the whole gamut of human experience, which was an education in itself for Chris, and he was always ready to enliven it with a witty rejoinder.

Needless to say, both Patrick and Hilary were deeply interested in Christopher's progress, helping where they could, although they were now living their own lives away from home. At about this time Hilary was given an opportunity to go to Nova Scotia, to help in the establishment of a small-holding in the depths of the beautiful Canadian forest. We were delighted that she was able to follow this dream, because one of our anxieties had always been that Christopher's accident might make Patrick and Hilary reluctant to follow their own careers without a feeling of guilt or restraint. Her letters, so full of poetic imagery, delighted Chris with their vivid descriptions of a life in which he was in such sympathy. She came home each Christmas, when the harshness of the Canadian winter would temporarily put an end to her horticultural activities; then her traveller's tales would give a new dimension to Christopher's circumscribed life.

Chapter Eleven

New Vistas

When I reflect on what Chris eventually achieved and how uni-que that achievement was, I am filled with pride. But none of this would have been possible without years of dedicated help given by so many dear friends. The teams of helpers continued the regular working sessions for over seven years. They gave not only their physical help (and that was a real struggle at times) but they also provided gaiety and fun; a joyousness lightened all the sessions giving us much needed relief from what could have been gruelling pressure. For those seven years our friends made their way to Gaterounds regardless of the weather and personal inconvenience, only their own domestic crises or a move away from the district interrupting their regular routine.

Perhaps this is the right place to describe the exercises we first devised in 1976 and the changes we made as they were gradually developed to adapt to full involvement by Chris. When we first started they were totally passive: Chris was un-able to help us in any way, although the very first hint of con-trolled movement had appeared about fifteen months after his accident. I have already described the first slight movements of his thumb for 'Yes' and 'No'. This was followed some weeks later by a weak hand-clasp; some movement of his right foot and toes was discernible at this time too. There had never been any sudden return to voluntary movement; it had always been a slowly developing subtle improvement of which I became aware long before others.

Gradually the impassivity of his appearance gave way to the

lop-sided expression of the hemiplegic as the muscles of his face developed, thus restoring some liveliness of expression, that had for so long been lacking. I also noticed that there was improvement in the colour and warmth of the skin on the right side of his body due to improved circulation, and that with this there was an increase in skin sensitivity, although the poor circulation and numbness of his left side remained unaltered for about five years of exercising. This meant that his left leg in particular had to be raised after only short periods of hanging low because it would swell and readily become blue. Adjustable leg rests fitted to his chair eased this problem.

When we had moved to Gaterounds he was quite unable to assist himself in any way. He had to be bolstered firmly in his wheelchair to prevent his falling out. His sense of balance was non-existent; he was incapable of holding his head up, and there was frequently a dribble from the right corner of his mouth. Five years after the accident he could still only swallow liquidized foods with difficulty and thinner fluids not at all. I was all too fearfully aware of how pathetic he must appear to strangers and how reserved and nervous they would be of approaching him. My natural inclination was to hide him from their gaze but I forced myself to suppress this, knowing that I should need help if any worthwhile life was going to be possible for him. Aware as I was of his mental strengths, I knew his physical abilities had to be developed to equal them. Otherwise his lively mind would be forever imprisoned in a helpless body, and its full expression would be rendered impossible.

So it was that we started the exercises in September 1976, the only interruptions to our regime occurring on the rare occasions when Chris was unwell. I read Glen Doman's book from cover to cover, and made detailed notes of the exercises he describes for children. Then I made a timetable of exercises to be carried out over a two hour period, this being the time I allotted, morning and evening, for each session. They were timed precisely, for I was determined to follow the directions to the letter although I realised that I might find that some of them would prove unsuitable for a full-grown adult.

The 'patterning' which Doman considered essential to the recovery of a brain-injured child was the imposition upon the child of movements that a normal child would instinctively use when learning to crawl. He believed that these exercises had to be done regularly, insistently and vigorously. We did five minutes of patterning eight times a day; and because Chris was an adult, it was necessary to use five helpers to carry this out properly, although for a small child only three are needed. Four of us would take one limb apiece, and the fifth was responsible for moving his head regularly from side to side as is done in the swimming crawl. The padded exercising pallet I had made was put on top of Chris' bed, and he was placed face downwards on it. It was important to make the movements in a regular, rhythmic manner; so these were often done to the rousing choruses of marching songs!

In the early years all his exercises were carried out on his bed because his condition was too delicate for him to be lifted on to the floor. His circulation was so poor that he could easily have become chilled, however warm we kept his room. But gradually his condition improved and he toughened. We used electrical vibrators to massage his entire body, hoping to stimulate his superficial circulation and improve the tone and sensitivity of his skin. This was most useful and eventually even the circulation to his left side became normal.

Soon after starting we noticed a marked improvement in his whole appearance, the dribble from his mouth disappeared and there was a general livening of the expression on his face: his eyes began to move in unison and developed a brightness that gave intelligence to his look. The flabbiness about his jaw line disappeared and his facial colour became more healthy. The more alert expression was enlivened by a wicked grin which we came to know so well over the years and which never failed to lift our hearts. Although physically he had changed, his character remained much the same old Chris, full of humour and kindness and very slow to anger.

His condition eventually was so much better that we were able to do most of his exercises on the floor which meant that we could extend their range. We were able to roll him over and over the length of the room in order to stimulate his sense of balance. Also we would help him to crawl across the floor, each of us taking a limb. To encourage him in this — for it really took a tremendous effort on his part — we would offer various enticements at journey's end: sometimes a fruit yoghurt, sometimes a can of beer but, most successfully, the prettiest girl available!

Gradually we extended his exercises. The equipment that we now needed to increase their scope was provided by the Department of Health and Social Security. They fitted a ceiling hoist which not only enabled me to get him in and out of the bath, but which I adapted to enable brachiation to be carried out. This is the American name given to an exercise to improve the capacity of the lungs — vital for tetraplegics because they are especially vulnerable to respiratory troubles. It consisted of raising Christopher's arms fully above his head and gradually moving him from the prone position on the floor to an upright sitting position. In this way not only was his breathing helped but his spine was stretched and made stronger.

Although in the early days Chris was unable to help himself at all, later he could hold the bar of the hoist with both his hands and actually participate in the entire exercise, only requiring me behind him in case he should slip. I tried out everything that had proved beneficial to the children whose case histories Glen Doman had published but, if I found that any of these exercises were not suitable for Chris after a reasonable trial, I discontinued them. One such exercise entailed hanging Chris by the feet from the ceiling. To accomplish this, an engineer friend had devised an ingenious contraption which operated by a pulley and rope attached to the hoist. It was very successful mechanically, but Chris soon became tired and felt sick. The idea was to stimulate his sense of balance, but we had to give it up. Exercises designed for young children are not necessarily satisfactory for a six foot, twelve-and-a-half-stone adult.

As he grew stronger and his abilities increased, albeit only weakly on his left side, we decided to use a standing bar. We would run his wheelchair up to a bar fixed across the door frame, then with his feet set squarely on a mat of foam rubber to prevent him from slipping, he would grip the bar with his right hand and pull himself into a standing position. His right side was very strong but he needed considerable help with his left hand hold. Ready helpers held his left arm and stood behind to give him support. The first time that he was able to rise to his feet by holding the bar alone, was thrilling to us all. He used to relish this accomplishment, just standing to gaze out of the window onto our lovely garden with the cows grazing in the meadow beyond.

Later we fixed a ladder across the ceiling of his room to help him to start taking the first steps towards our eventual aim of independent walking. With his left arm round my shoulders and my arm about his waist to support him, he would grip the rungs of the ladder above his head with his right hand. Then he was able to step forward naturally and strongly with his right leg, though his left leg needed help from my foot to be moved forward. In the course of time, he would step forward with his left leg too, and when he did this it was with the same controlled and purposeful movement as with his right. Although he still required my support, he was now holding himself much more upright and he would sometimes in this way step right across the room.

About ten years after his accident it was evident that function was slowly returning to the whole of his left side in the same way that we had earlier noted with his right side. I likened these slow developments to the rising of the sap in a tree in springtime. Strengthening movement developed from his fingers up his arms and from his toes and feet up his legs to his trunk.

His exercises became more and more active: he was no longer a mere passive recipient; rather, he participated fully and was able to make at least some contribution to every exercise. Some of my helpers who were judo enthusiasts suggested that we incorporated some of their exercises in the sessions, particularly those relating to body movement. Chris became proficient in these and took a delight in exceeding their efforts. He was able to arch his back higher than any of us. Arm and leg movements were adapted and he became accomplished at swinging his hips — we used to call this 'the John Travolta exercise'. By this time he was actively exercising every muscle in his body; although some movements were still only very weak, with a bit of help all were eventually possible to him.

Increasingly he was able to help me with the different movements that were required for his day-to-day management. He could arch his back and move himself across the bed to adjust his position; he could roll over, pulling himself to the side of the bed, and swing his legs across the bed and over the side. He was able to help take his shirt and jersey off. His balance was tremendously improved and he no longer sagged in a chair but could pull himself upright. As his back muscles grew stronger and his balance improved, he would pull himself forward to the edge of his seat and with his arms firmly round my neck would raise himself to a standing position; then, turning he would be able to sit down in another chair. This was a blessing since it enabled him easily to change from his wheelchair to an easy chair in our lounge, something he particularly liked to do for watching television. All the time he was learning to do this with less and less hold on my shoulders, taking more of his weight on his own two feet. We both of us felt that the day was approaching when he would be able to stand up alone. We sensed that we were on the home stretch.

Anyone unaccustomed to dealing with a severely disabled person might have considered that Christopher's improvements were sorely restricted and inadequate. But in the context of the prolonged period of unconsciousness he had suffered and his total helplessness over so many years, his slow return of function and the measure of independence he gained was truly astonishing. In due course he could feed himself on our normal meals, using a spoon single-handed; he could drink what he liked without choking; he could communicate by writing and even his speech began to come back, though slowly. It was wonderful that that most human of attributes was returning to help him towards normality.

He was always of an independent spirit, and it was the acquiring of communicative skills that made the greatest difference to his quality of life. The very first form of communication that he used was the thumb movement, up and down for *yes* and *no*. Then, within the year, of his own volition, he developed finger writing on his chest, always writing the letters the right way round for the viewer. Later he began to use a pencil and pad; for a long time his hand needed help across the page, but with improved muscular control his writing became clearer.

His speech started to return very weakly at first — just the faintest whisper deep down in his throat — but that too gradually became stronger and clearer. I constantly had to remind him to articulate more clearly and accentuate his consonants, especially the final ones. But he suffered no block to word use: he could express himself exactly as he wished to. He always chose his words precisely, with subtle usage and correct syntax, delighting in their beauty. Indeed it was a speciality of his to construct long, complex, rounded sentences, rather than to settle for a telegraphese that might have made conversation a rather more speedy process.

Comprehension was no difficulty whatsoever; we could speak to him in the most rapid and sophisticated manner on matters of any complexity, without having to make any concessions to him at all. This new found freedom of communication was a blessing to him, enabling him to establish a true rapport with his friends and helpers. He could be relied upon to contribute a witty and original comment whatever the subject might be. He would pick up a passing remark in a trice and flash back with a most apposite comment.

There were times when he would mischievously take advantage of a situation of momentary quiet, making an outspoken comment that might have been better left unsaid. He was never one to avoid a good Anglo-Saxon expression if he felt things were getting a trifle too precious and if anyone questioned his use of a robust four-lettered word, he would declare that he was studying for his 'A' levels in that subject! This was so like the old Chris, it was a joy to behold.

During our often boisterous and always merry sessions our talk used to range from the serious to the ridiculous. We had tremendous fun acting the fool with him or engaging in serious philosophical argument; we were continually surprised by his sharpness of wit and his capacity for original and wry comment about some event. He had a lovely sense of humour, never malicious, always kind. It was an agony to him if he thought someone's feelings had been hurt.

He used to enjoy thought-provoking games about words, pursuing their associations and different meanings and working out their derivations. He loved doing intelligence tests, especially about scientific formulae, dates, authors, geography, botany and birds. His memory for such things was excellent and he would take a delight in outshining his helpers, who would give in with a good grace, tongue in cheek, to his 'superior intelligence', as they would say!

He had wide interests and catholic tastes, and was never a boring companion. He was fond of music; his favourite instrument was the violin, which he had once started to learn. He had a sensitive ear for the lyrical and poignant: Tchaikovsky, Mahler, Ravel and Grieg were among his favourites. He loved the voices of Kathleen Ferrier and Kiri Te Kanawa, always choosing to listen to their tapes if he was feeling unwell or in need of comfort. Poetry would restore him, especially the poems of Dylan Thomas. He loved long narrative verse like *Hiawatha* and the *First Settler's Story.* Masefield's *Sea Fever* was always a favourite. Art gave him endless delight: we would spend happy hours perusing our books of Picasso, Van Gogh, Claude Monet and the British landscape painters. We took him to London in his wheelchair to see the exhibitions of Constable paintings at the Tate Gallery and Turner at the Royal Academy, gaining access through diverse gates and lifts thanks to the kindness of elderly commissionaires. He had a special feeling for George Stubbs' animal studies, his interest in biology and taxidermy giving him a respect for Stubbs' interpretation of animal form and movement.

Radio and television programmes provided him with many interests. Although he was a discriminating listener and viewer, he had favourites amongst all types of programmes — natural history, Esther Rantzen's *That's Life,* or *Dad's Army.* He loved televised orchestral concerts, especially those conducted by André Prévin, whose informal style suited Chris' easy going ways. The Last Night of the Proms was an annual highlight.

Notwithstanding the shattering blow that had so nearly destroyed him, his was, in its way, an involved and interested life. He was aware of his achievements and was proud of them.

A friend asked me if I ever lost my temper with Chris; one can get cross with those nearest and dearest, most especially when under a prolonged strain. After his accident I honestly don't believe I did. Certainly in the past, while bringing up the children, I had got exasperated and lost my temper on occasion, but it was rare and not lasting — just the normal quick flare-up when you feel exasperated beyond reason. In the circumstances I have been describing, when I was working with the injured Chris, I knew that he was always trying his best, if he didn't work as I wished it was because he was not well. I simply could not have lost my temper with him — I was too aware of his immense patience and courage.

Chapter Twelve

A Serious Setback

Christopher's story has brought us up to the early summer of 1980, nearly eleven years after his accident. After the trauma, turmoil and the complete disruption of all our lives over the previous decade, it might be felt that at least we would now be left to pursue our chosen course in peace and some degree of equanimity. In no way was this to be so. Once more, out of a tranquil sky, came shattering disaster.

I had realised for some time that Christopher's teeth were in serious need of attention, but it had proved impossible to get anyone to undertake this locally. By this time Paddy had qualified as a doctor. He was a Registrar at the Royal Free Hospital at Hampstead in north London, and was able to interest his medical and dental colleagues in his brother's problem. After examining Chris as an out-patient, the dentists decided that the work needed was so extensive that it would have to be carried out under a general anaesthetic. So it was decided to admit Chris to hospital for two or three days. Before leaving home he was put onto a course of antibiotic to reduce the risk of infection, and on the appointed day, 1st June, we travelled across London in Dobbin to the hospital.

As I waited for Chris to return from the operating theatre, I became increasingly anxious. I was allowed into the recovery room to be with him as he came round from the anaesthetic. It was soon apparent that he was having serious breathing difficulty. As hour succeeded hour without his recovering consciousness it became clear that he had suffered post-operative respiratory failure. He was in a coma, but this time totally dependent on a mechanical respirator. He was taken from the operating theatre to the Intensive Therapy Unit and once again we were at his bedside, watching him fighting for his life.

Although we had known that there was a considerable risk inherent in the operation, we were not prepared for a disaster on this scale. It was a shattering blow to us all, but further, I felt desperately sorry for the people who had helped to arrange this essential treatment. It is extremely difficult to obtain dental care for a disabled person and for this grave complication to have arisen must have been dreadfully distressing to the staff concerned. Most especially I grieved for Paddy. Since qualifying he had specialised in anaesthesia and it is the doctors of this discipline who are responsible for the Intensive Therapy Units in hospitals. His experience following Chris' original accident had led him to a special interest in the care of such critically ill people and he has developed particular skill and understanding in this field of medicine. Although he had not been involved in the operation, it hardly seemed credible that such an ironic twist of fate should lead to his brother now struggling for his life in his own unit in his own hospital.

Over the next few days Christopher gradually recovered consciousness but all attempts to wean him off the respiratory machine failed. Each day that passed compounded the seriousness of his situation, but there were two essential differences between this occasion and the first one of over ten years earlier. One was that he was conscious, although once again completely helpless and unable to communicate; the other was that I was at peace. Despite the sorrow and anxiety which I felt in my mind, my heart was at peace. It was as though for the first time I was able to understand the true meaning of the phrase in the Lord's Prayer, 'Thy will be done'. I felt a quiet acceptance that, whatever the outcome, it would be right for Chris.

I had been given a private room at the hospital so as to be near him, and I received every kindness and thoughtful attention from the medical and nursing staff. I was treated as a colleague and a friend. Although he lay once more attached to, and surrounded by, the horrifying tubes and electronic equipment of modern medicine, as far as possible I worked with Chris. I felt cold fear at the sight of all this paraphernalia and had a doomed sense of history repeating itself. It seemed as though Fate, having been cheated once, was determined not to let the quarry slip a second time. Yet, despite all this, I was astonished to find I remained calm. Quietly taking up once more the work I had devised so many years before, I began the persistent rubbing and soft talk which I believed would give him reassurance and comfort, massaging his arms and hands and softly speaking of much loved things.

For the first time since his accident I was not continually busy and I had time to think. My paradoxical attitude seemed inexplicable to me and I tried hard to understand it. *Knowing so certainly* what I had to do, I was able to consider the intervening years dispassionately. Slowly it dawned on me that the secret of my changed attitude lay in that very certainty. Now I was not distressed by a sense of guilt, almost betrayal. At the moment of Christopher's greatest need I had not withdrawn myself and left to others what I felt in my heart should be my own responsibility. Through the years I had been shown a way to follow. I knew how the bond of love could be used as a vital weapon, in conjunction with skilled medical attention, to bring comfort. Whether Chris lived or died, I knew that I was able to give him this last service that our mutual love demanded. It is a natural loving rite that our human condition requires and one denied to so many people in a social environment in which advanced medical methods demand that the seriously ill are taken away from their home surroundings and loved ones into the starkly alien world of the hospital. It is not the will that is lacking but the knowledge of how these two essential needs may be reconciled to mutual advantage that requires still to be understood.

Birth and death are natural events: it is how one deals with them that is important. In more primitive cultures there is a ritual and a caring within the family structure which both prepares the family for bereavement and helps the dying. In the England of Victorian times, death was a more frequent visitor to the larger families of those days. I do not believe it was any numbing of the sense of loss caused by repeated blows that enabled them to accept bereavement more easily than we do today. Rather, I think it was the opportunity that their different lifestyle afforded them to use their love in their family surroundings to comfort and support their dear ones, which eased their mourning. The Victorian sick-room, like the open fireplace, had a therapy to offer: by discarding them in favour of what seems to be material advance, we are in fact diminished and impoverished.

Today an unacknowledged sense of guilt often compounds the distress of death. The advanced technology of medicine is wonderful and must be used to the full, but I hope the message inherent in Christopher's story, of the vital contribution that love can make, will show that this too can be used as an essential tool.

The intensive care units of our major hospitals are centres of excellence to which people of all nationalities and backgrounds are drawn, brought together by overriding love and the desire to be near their dear ones at the time of their greatest need. It is not just the appalling ever-rising toll of road accidents that fills these units, there is also a never-ending stream of cardiac arrest and stroke cases, brain-damaged victims of terrorism and violence, and perhaps surprisingly, especially in America, swimming pool accident cases. Those who, at a moment's notice, find themselves keeping vigil for their loved ones in these bleak clinical rooms are often tormented by a deep sense of helplessness and fear which increases their anguish. Suddenly I realised that by sharing Christopher's story with the sorrowing relatives amongst whom I found myself in the waiting room, I could show them that they had a job to do: one that only *they* were capable of doing and which would be uniquely comforting, whatever the outcome of their ordeal.

It was wonderful to see the relief flood their faces. The local chemist in Hampstead sold out of the fresheners which I had recommended as an aid to the gentle massaging, so we made our own from lint and eau de cologne. Thus I was able to witness the inspiration which the lessons learnt through the long years of working with Chris was able to give. The withdrawn misery was changed, as if by alchemy, to a shared sympathy and sense of purpose.

One example of the comfort which this wrought was touching and unforgettable. An old lady was admitted, deeply unconscious following a stroke. Her husband was a London Eastender of the cockney sparrow type, well into his eighties; they were a true Darby and Joan. He was brought to the hospital each day by a kind young man who shared his vigil. Once there the old man would sit withdrawn in the waiting room, stunned by the shocking event.

I found it agonising to watch his misery, so I told him how I thought he could help his wife, and how he must speak to her about familiar things. He bought some eau de cologne fresheners, but his relief quickly turned to consternation: what could he talk to her about? Through the long years of their married life they had developed a silent understanding with little need of conversation! Desperately I tried to discover some subject of mutual interest, but to no avail. They had no children, no cat or dog, not even a garden. There seemed to be nothing of sufficient interest to sustain a soliloquy of love. So I told him he would have to reach back into the memories of their courting days: these would surely be etched deeply into his Annie's mind.

So he set to work, and after a rather shaky start I was overjoyed to see him massaging his wife's arm and animatedly talking to her. Later, I learnt from his young man companion that they shared a mutual devotion to horse racing. It was no reminiscing of young love that we were seeing, but a subject of almost equal passion. What the young man heard was 'I say old girl, d'you know who won the Derby? young Willie Carson on *Henbit*, they romped home by a length . . . seven to one!'

His dear old Dutch died, but her memory will live with me forever. I know the sadness of her husband's loss will have been eased by the knowledge that when she needed him most he was there beside her giving his love. In the ensuing weeks so many people passed through the waiting room, and a very special and deeply comforting bond of friendship was developed between us, born out of our common concern and shared sympathy. Their stay was usually brief: either their loved one died, or recovered sufficiently to be transferred to the normal wards.

Only Chris remained: each attempt to take him off his respirator and oxygen supply precipitated a crisis. Above all, he had to be protected against anoxaemia and consequent further brain damage, which could set at nought everything that had been gained through the years. Guy, Paddy and I (Hilary was in Canada) were faced with the ultimate awesome question that any family can ever be asked: if it was in our power, *would* we switch off that respirator? While Chris was conscious, this would not be asked of us, but if his condition deteriorated, we had to know what our decision would be. How we longed to have him home where all the decisions would once more be in our own hands. But we were unanimous in our thoughts that the only thing of importance to Chris was the quality of his life, not its length.

Then, towards the end of the third week, the consultant who had Chris in her care felt that the dilatory respiratory centre in his brain was reasserting itself just sufficiently to make the risk of taking him off the respirator acceptable. On the twenty first day after his operation this was accomplished and we were told that if he did not deteriorate over the next forty-eight hours then, precarious though his condition might still be, we could take him home.

Discharging a patient direct from the Intensive Therapy Unit in this way was unprecedented, and it was a measure of the consultant's recognition of the uniqueness of the situation. Chris held his ground and on the second day Guy brought Dobbin to the hospital. Touchingly the unit staff, whom we had come to appreciate so much, gathered to say goodbye and wish him well — such dear faces from the Caribbean, the Far East, Ireland and the shires of England. With thankfulness but also with a desperate anxiety that some further complication might prevent our getting away at the last minute, we set off across central London for home.

Strangely, from that moment onwards Chris went from strength to strength. The setback had been serious, forcing us to revert once more to the constant nursing and chest therapy of the early days for several weeks after his homecoming. But before very long his physical abilities were restored to their previous level, and then his slow but steady progress was re-established. Another milestone had been passed on the extraordinary journey that Christopher had been called on to make. As we have accompanied him on his journey, Guy and I have constantly been borne up by the words of Arthur Hugh Clough:

> *Say not the struggle nought availeth . . .*
> *. . . For while the tired waves, vainly breaking,*
>   *Seem here no painful inch to gain,*
> *Far back, through creeks and inlets making,*
>   *Comes silent, flooding in the main . . .*

Chapter Thirteen

The Buttercup Summer

And so to 1983, one of the most beautiful years I can remember. Day followed day bringing clear skies, sunshine and warm soft breezes, reminding me of the hot dreamy days of my youth, which we used to call 'buttercup summers'. Spring was cold and wet, but this seemed only to increase the rich blossoming that followed. Hitherto reluctant plants flowered for the first time: our garden was alive with bees, and butterflies came to our lavender in great numbers, among them species that we had long thought lost. Chris had never enjoyed the garden so much. All day and every day he was outside, either over in the farmyard or in a shady spot on the lawn.

All our cows calved in the spring, with enough milk for each to foster two more as well. There was nothing that gave Chris greater pleasure than to watch the birth of a calf and then to witness the always wondrous phenomenon of mother and calf bonding. He would insist on staying out to watch the birth, however delayed it might be, even though darkness had fallen. There then followed the challenging and fascinating process of persuading the mother to accept and foster a further two newly-born calves, which we would obtain by telephoning round friends and neighbours who had surplus calves from dairy herds. In due course the day would come to release the suckler herd in the fields.

This was a glorious moment, an entrancingly natural and lovely sight of which we could never tire: seven cows with twenty-one calves all running and skipping and cavorting with the sudden release of the pent-up spirits of winter. Our beautiful home-bred bull, a splendid Hereford, was named Sir Thomas Beecham — all our cows had been given musical names. Our first cow had been a gift and happened to be called Lyric, and this started the theme. We had some difficulty in choosing musical names that would not sound too strange, but we ended up with cows called Melody, Madrigal, Polonaise, Minuet, Rhapsody, Minstrel and Allegro, with two young heifers, Song and Calypso. So that Chris should feel as closely involved in our farming operation as was possible, we had hand reared all these from a few days old, so that they were perfectly tame and manageable. These great beasts, which can appear so daunting to the uninitiated, have in fact gentle placid natures, and are so easy to handle.

Our meadows were ancient permanent grassland, with all the beautiful multiplicity of grasses and herbs that this implies. We managed this by rotational grazing, rolling and harrowing, and manuring with farmyard manure from our winter yard, using a vintage tractor and a manure spreader. Chris would come into the fields in his electric Batricar, and from a safe and shady place would keep his eye on the unpaid farm labourer — his mother! What fun we had. Every day we would take our meals wherever we were working, usually joined by Jane, our sheep dog, Ra, our Abyssinian cat and our flock of Muscovy ducks. These had started the summer as one duck and drake, but five ducklings later, the seven would follow us, trailing behind wherever we went; Chris decided that the collective term we should use was a *ribbon* of ducks!

It was a fruitful year. We collected fresh raspberries, gooseberries, and later, blackberries from the hedgerows, and apples from our orchard. Chris had the eye of an artist and was quick to see beauty in all things great and small in the natural world. This year I think the splendid Turneresque sunsets caught his imagination more than anything else. Evening after evening he would sit out in the balmy air with the sky changing from amber to scarlet, the sun slowly sinking behind the silhouetted

line of chestnut trees on the western skyline beyond our cattle
yard. Satisfied that the red sky had assured us of another lovely
day, he would watch the moon and stars appear, only agreeing
to come in to bed when I had threatened to go to bed before
him.

Although he spent most of each day outside, we persisted
with his exercises. Each morning three friends would arrive to
carry out the taxing regime. By this time Chris was making a
considerable contribution to every exercise: they were no longer
passive, and could be decidedly lively. If he considered that we
were a little lukewarm in our praise he would tell us reproach-
fully that he considered he had made a 'bloody fine effort'!
Sometimes, if he was feeling disinclined to work and felt that
we should leave him in peace, we would be told in no uncertain
terms what he thought of us. Mainly, however, he enjoyed working at his exercises; he was delighted by his achievements,
taking pride in the return of his strength and abilities. Of course
the pretty young women were appreciated, but he also had an
eye for the more mature charms of some of the older helpers,
while with the young men he had a particular and racy rapport.
What friendship his helpers gave him and how he loved them!

The delightful summer of 1983 passed into an equally beautiful autumn, a veritable Indian summer. On 5th October Chris
had been out with me as usual, as I worked in the cattle yard
with the tractor, shifting out the old straw bedding to prepare it
for bringing the cows in for the winter. Our two young heifers,
his special pets, were in the enclosure with him, while our dog
and cat and all the ducks were at his feet. It was a pastoral scene
of gentle beauty that will never fade from my mind. Towards
evening he complained of feeling tired so I brought him in a little earlier than usual. Guy was mowing the lawn, the sweet
smell of the cut grass hanging on the air. Chris, stopping his
electrically-propelled chair, suddenly insisted on Guy turning
round. There, for all to see, the seam of his trousers was split up
the back, revealing a strip of white cotton underpants! Un-

beknown to his father, Chris had seen him as he was pulling the starter-cord of the lawnmower and had seen the trousers split. How he laughed, such a happy joyous sound!

And so he came in and went to bed. Usually he would watch television with us, but this particular night: he simply said he was too tired. This worried me a little because Guy had recently recovered from a sharp virus infection, and I had feared it might affect Chris and me. However, once he was in bed he said he felt fine and would like his supper. He was always so grateful for whatever I did for him, and would call the simplest meal delicious. This evening he'd apologised to me for not being sociable and feeling flopped, so I settled him down to sleep earlier than usual.

Next morning as I was preparing him for his exercises, I thought he was being a little slow and asked him how he felt. 'Proper poorly' was his reply with a disarming grin, so I decided when his helpers arrived that we would let him rest. Instead we all turned our energies to finishing cleaning out the cattle yard, people coming in to have a word with Chris at frequent intervals. He thoroughly enjoyed this attention, but as the day wore on I realised he was becoming a bit chesty and was developing a temperature. It was not that that he was obviously ill, but because Guy had been ill, this made me anxious. So I decided to sleep downstairs with him, as was my custom when he was not well.

Whenever he was unwell he loved to have a sentimental loving goodnight and to be reminded of the family, how much we all loved him and how proud of him we were. Hilary had written one of her long descriptive letters from Nova Scotia which had arrived only that morning, and I read this to him. He was so touchingly sweet, somehow so vulnerable: he kept squeezing my hand and I in return put my fond kisses in his. I asked him if he would like me to sleep on the floor beside his bed, as I had done so often in the past, but he said that it would be all right if I slept in the next room with the doors left open.

Later Guy looked in to say goodnight to Chris and see how he was. He told me some time later that Chris had reached out to take his hand and would scarcely let it go, giving the African reversed handshake that they often used as a secret thing between them. Then Chris gave him that dazzling smile that could pierce your heart, and Guy just put his arms round him and hugged him and kissed him and whispered, 'Dear God take care of you'.

Before he went upstairs to bed Guy and I discussed Chris' condition: we agreed that he was only the same as he had been on several occasions in the past when influenza-like infections were going round, and we decided that we would only call our doctor if we were not happy about him in the morning.

So we both went to bed, but of course I did not sleep. Through the years I had developed a resting alert state that any slight change in his condition could instantly arouse. Throughout the night I went into his room at intervals to watch him, and each time I found him in a relaxed and peaceful sleep, quietly and comfortably breathing.

Then, just after sunrise, at about seven o'clock, I became aware of a strangely complete silence, a holy quiet. I rose from my bed and went in to his room. Chris had simply stopped breathing. A radiance lit his face: he looked more vibrantly alive than I had seen him for years. Peacefully, without anxiety or struggle, he had left us. The last stitches of our precious son's tapestry had been finished. I called Guy, and with our arms round each other and round Chris we wept silently.

Christopher's death was sudden and unexpected, leaving a gap in many lives in our village. For eight years through all weathers, winter and summer, our helpers had made their way to Gaterounds to help with his exercises. The members of each team had become such a loyal band of friends, each group with a distinctive character of its own; he was loved and admired by them all. But as so often when bread is cast upon the waters, it is returned to you in unexpected ways. I believe that Christopher's room and our daily meetings there became valuable to our helpers in their own lives; for, as we worked, we talked and in this way personal problems and worries were informally broached and tossed about; anxieties were eased and much wisdom and experience passed to and fro. In short, our groups became centres of psychological therapy of a most practical and valuable kind. The thread that ran through this process was Chris' staunch over-riding of his personal tragedy.

After his death, apart from telling us of their sadness at losing a dear friend, the almost universal comment was that the inspiration of his courage would be with them always and would sustain them through any trials that they too might have to face. The memory of his original wit and lovely sense of humour brings laughter to any company of his friends. After his funeral at the village church most of them returned to our house, and it was a time for happy remembering, despite the heartbreak we felt.

Christopher was buried amongst the yew trees in the graveyard of our beautiful 800-year-old parish church. As we laid him quietly to rest in the soft autumn rain, only our family and a few very old friends stood round his grave, for we wished the service that was to follow in the church to be a thanksgiving for his life. The church was packed full; there were old schoolfriends, and friends from our Hertfordshire days, all so faithful in their remembrance, troubling to come so far; family friends, close relatives, old and young, and so many of our village friends were there to give us comfort and support. We found it impossible to express our thankfulness in words; we just gave them our hearts. It was the very evocation of Joyce Grenfell's poem, *To sing as well*.

Chris loved music and poetry, and we chose hymns that were either his favourite pieces, or which spoke to us of his splendid qualities. While we were gathered round his grave we could hear the soft strains of a Bach anthem being played to the people waiting in the church, and as we came in to join them, this changed to 'Jesu, joy of man's desiring'. The congregation sang 'The Lord is my shepherd', followed by John Bunyan's pilgrim's hymn 'He who would true valour see'; and finally, as we knelt, our village choir sang as an anthem 'God be in my heart'. Patrick read the lesson, and the prayers were led by our constant friend and supporter, Reverend Phipps-Jones. The following extract comes from the address given by our rector, Dennis Parker:

'What shall we say of these fourteen years since Chris' terrible accident? I am not trying to be clever when I use an unusual word, but one that for me expresses in an adequate way what has happened during these long and sometimes sad and trying years. It is the word, known to scientists, 'kinetic'. When I began my training in industry and I was at the outset put in the laboratory before being released into the works, ultimately to represent my company, I had to learn what kinetic energy meant. Simply, kinetic energy is the energy possessed by a body by virtue of its motion. Thus we say that almost every object has this potential . . . a stone possesses it, in that it can roll down a slope. It does not develop the energy when it is still, but once it has the conditions in which motion is possible, then it moves, releasing its kinetic energy.

I hope that is a correct use of the word — for in these fourteen years we have witnessed something of the kinetic energy of a community . . . the potential for love and kindness that is often unrealised until some event, some great need, some tragedy calls for that potential; we have seen a large group of volunteers joining with Christopher's family, and applying love, patience, zeal and support in order to regain for Chris a reasonable measure of existence. Those kindnesses — that spiritual kinetic energy — comes from the Lord; just as man's sin arises from our inbred self-centredness, so kindness, goodness, care and concern come from His grace working in our lives. All of us regret Chris' death . . . and yet these years have not been wasted, and when looked back on from the perspective of the future, they will be seen as years full of all that makes life worthwhile; all that makes society beneficial; years speaking of the grace of God.'

The other day a dear friend suggested that it would be helpful if I tried to define my faith. She knew of Christopher's accident and how my belief in God's help had sustained me through the long years of working with him. I find it as impossible to describe as the air I breathe, and as vital to my life. Jesus told us that God is love, and I believe that Jesus was God incarnate — a friend in whom I can trust implicitly. If I pray with all my heart and work with all my strength, I believe that guidance will be granted to me, remembering always, 'Not my will, but thine, Lord'.

Christopher's accident did not strengthen or change my faith, it simply confirmed it. There is evil as well as good in this world, there is sinning and redemption, courage and cowardice, hope and despair; everything has its opposite. Nothing, I believe, can withstand the power of pure goodness which is the love of God, but man has the awesome freedom to choose. I don't pretend to be a theologian; I only know that for me the love of God is the essence of life.

A few days after Chris' death, as I was sadly clearing up his room, I came across his writing pad on which I had left him to write his thoughts as I was working in the farmyard on that last day. He had grown tired towards the late afternoon and so I had brought him in and put him to bed without looking to see what had been written. Did he have some premonition of what was so soon to follow? For on the paper, written with unusual clarity, were the simple words, *Myrtle, I love you.* This was his expression of what our years together had meant to him, and this was his last loving goodbye to me.

The Buttercup Summer

It was on my birthday, Friday 7th October 1983, at first light, that Chris left us. I believe that he and I had reached the sunny uplands we had kept in our sights for so long.

Strangely, Christopher's death from an overwhelming chest infection was probably very like that of a climber suffering from a lack of oxygen in the rarefied air of the high mountains. He could have died in no quieter nor more gentle way. Hypoxaemia in such conditions is a curiously relaxed, even euphoric state, with dreams of home and friends, and a sense of the rightness of things filling the mind, while one drifts in and out of consciousness. I believe that this is how Chris died; slipping into death gently, it came to him as a welcoming friend. We could not look upon his serenely beautiful face and radiant smile that morning without knowing it was God's last gift to him.

But we, being human, miss him most dreadfully. The world seems an empty place without him, and parting is hell, as Joyce Grenfell has written:

> *If I should go before the rest of you,*
> *Break not a flower nor inscribe any stone.*
> *Nor, when I'm gone speak in a Sunday voice,*
> *But be yourselves that I have known.*
> > *Weep if you must,*
> > *Parting is hell,*
> > *But life goes on,*
> > *So sing as well.*

She expresses perfectly what is in my heart. It is because 'life goes on' that I have written this story. Chris was essentially a practical person and he would have scorned the proposition that, because one member of the expedition had become a casualty, the rest should not press on. He was always a leader, innovator and improviser. The Africans have an embracing word to describe these qualities; it is *hodari*. Chris would have been proud to be called *hodari Yeoman*!

It was with infinite patience and unique talent that he was able to put together the shattered fragments of his life, creating a work of such beauty, inspiration and delight that those of us left behind, who were privileged to know his companionship and love, count ourselves blessed.